A Race for Life

A Race for Life

A Diet and Exercise Program for Superfitness
and Reversing the Aging Process

*The amazing story of how one woman
survived breast cancer to take on the
toughest races in the world*

RUTH E. HEIDRICH, PH.D.

LANTERN PUBLISHING & MEDIA • BROOKLYN, NY

2020
Lantern Publishing & Media
128 Second Place
Brooklyn, NY 11231
www.lanternpm.org

This title was previously published by Booklight Inc. (DBA Lantern Books). In December 2019, Booklight Inc. transferred all its assets, including this book, to Lantern Publishing & Media, a new company dedicated to the same publishing mission as Lantern Books. Lantern Publishing & Media's printing of this book remains the same as the Lantern Books' version, unless otherwise indicated.

Printed in the United States of America

Library of Congress Cataloging-in-Publication Data

Heidrich, Ruth.
    A race for life : a diet and exercise program for superfitness and reversing the aging process : the amazing story of how one woman survived breast cancer to take on the toughest races in the world / by Ruth E. Heidrich.
        p. cm.
    Includes bibliographical references and index.
    ISBN 1-930051-00-X (alk. paper)
        1. Health. 2. Physical fitness. 3. Nutrition. 4. Heidrich, Ruth—Health. 5. Breast—Cancer—Patients—Hawaii—Biography. I. Title.

RA776 .H465 2000
613.7—dc21

00-025068

Contents

Contents

This book is dedicated to all who are interested in improving the quality of their lives. May you forever avoid the scourge of heart disease, cancer, stroke, diabetes, arthritis, osteoporosis, hypertension, obesity, and all the other diseases influenced by diet and exercise.

Acknowledgments

Writing this book has turned out to be an incredible adventure. I could never have done it without the support of some wonderful people. John A. McDougall, M.D., was the physician who turned my life around by educating me about my cancer. He also followed my progress as a volunteer subject in his breast cancer research.

Dr. McDougall was the first to suggest that I write a book about what I learned on this medical journey, saying that it would be of value to others. He believed in me enough to literally take me by the hand to a computer store where he showed me the wonders of computers and word processing. He then started a phone campaign, calling me to check up on my progress, assuring me that it was easy, "once you get started." Dr. McDougall was right. Writing this book was easy, but that's only from this vantage point. Looking at it from the beginning, it seemed nearly impossible.

As I increased my exercise, I ran into resistance from people who thought that I, as a cancer patient, should be "taking it easy." As my "unorthodox" medical program gained more attention, I started to get some publicity. This led to an appearance on "The Hour Magazine" with host, Gary Collins. On that show I got to tell the "whole world" about Kenneth Cooper, M.D. and how he launched me on my exercise program. Dr. Cooper, with his landmark book on aerobic exercise, altered my life forever, too.

Next, John Kay came into my life. He'd read my story in the Hawaii publication, *Midweek*. After he introduced himself to me, he asked if I'd ever considered writing a book. I told him that, by chance, I'd just started seriously considering it. He volunteered to help; and help he did. We met weekly for him to review the previous week's painful efforts. (Writing is easy; you just sit down at a typewriter and open a vein!) He critiqued my writing, patted me on the back, and sent me off to write some more.

Terry Shintani, M.D., entered the scene by giving me the opportunity to be co-host of a weekly, two-hour radio talk show, "Nutrition and You." We've been on the air for well over ten years now on every Sunday night. Working with Dr. Shintani has been invaluable, as he has given me support both as a physician and a friend. We've had some fabulous guests on our show and I have learned a lot. I really owe Bonnie Choy, RN, Bob Leitch, Bill Harris, M.D., Carl Weisbrod, Ph.D., Katie Payne, and a host of others. With inspiration and support like that, there may be more people who inspire me. The journey's far from over.

Foreword

For several years now, both medical and physical evidence has pointed to diet, exercise, and emotional factors as contributing in great measure today to the prevention of cancer, as well as some rather miraculous remissions and, in some cases, outright cures.

Ruth Heidrich tells a fascinating story of her progression from a woman devastated by the thought of losing her breast and, quite possibly, her life because of cancer to becoming an internationally recognized athlete.

Ruth's story needs to be told—not to glorify her athletic prowess, which is a story in itself—but to demonstrate there is a mix of diet, exercise, and mental conditioning that any one of us can use to fight the invasion of disease and depression in a natural way.

As the medical profession, coaches, and nutritionists gather evidence for our future benefit, people like Ruth Heidrich are at the forefront, proving that the way to a healthier, happier life and the prevention of disease are here today.

Terry Shintani, M.D., J.D., M.P.H.
Author of *Eat More, Weigh Less* and *The Hawaii Diet*

Diagnosis

The words "infiltrating ductal carcinoma" shocked and then numbed me. I could not believe what I had just heard. As the impact of that potential death sentence began to sink in, wild and uncontrollable panic seized me. "Oh, no!" I cried, "Oh, no, no...." The devastating words of the diagnosis of cancer echoed in my head as I fought back dizziness and nausea. I felt I was in some horrible nightmare from which I was about to awake.

Just minutes before, while waiting to hear the results of the biopsy from the pathology lab, I had been sure—in fact, certain—that the offending growth was benign. I kept telling myself that everything was going to be just fine—just like it had always been every other time in my life when tragedy threatened. Hadn't I always done everything I was supposed to? As the reality sank in, I felt totally alone. No one heard my silent scream, "This is not fair!"

I'd always eaten a "well-balanced" diet and had even sworn off red meat years before. I'd gotten plenty of exercise and, in fact, had even run marathons. I'd had frequent medical check-ups that included regular mammograms and had religiously examined my breasts every month.

How could this have happened? And why to me? Things like this happen only in movies—or to other people, I thought. I'd always led a relatively conventional life—healthy, successful, always playing by the rules. I'd even been dealt a good hand in the game of life, attractive enough to win a few beauty contests and have three appearances in the TV series, "Hawaii 5-O." I was well educated, held an engrossing, well-paying job as a GS-13 military logistician that involved traveling all over the world. All four grandparents had lived to the ripe old age of ninety, so I knew I had some pretty good genes. I had what I thought was a good, solid marriage and two bright, beautiful, and successful children. My life could not have been better!

So why this avalanche of devastation? It was both a life and a death sentence for me. It was a "life" sentence because there's still no real cure for breast cancer and a "death" sentence because breast cancer is a major killer of adult women, striking one out of every seven or eight American women. It happened also to be the number one killer of women in my age group.

"My God, what do I do now?" I asked the two surgeons who were attending me. "More surgery," the senior surgeon said. "I'd recommend a modified radical mastectomy since the tumor was so large."

I'd talked the surgeons into letting me watch the first operation (against their better judgment, they said). Instead of general anesthesia, I had had only a local anesthetic, and, therefore, had witnessed the surgeons carving a chunk the size of a golf ball out of my right breast. Thinking that I surely must be exaggerating the size of the mass in my mind, I kept trying to diminish the image. No, it was still horribly big, no matter how I visualized it.

The type of surgery the doctors now recommended would remove the breast tissue that remained after the biopsy, the fascia covering the chest muscles, the skin covering the breast area, the nipple, and all the lymph nodes in the axilla, or armpit. A lumpectomy was out of the question because there were cancer cells beyond all the margins of the tissue sample. The surgeons told me that, after the surgery, there would be tests to determine the spread. As it turned out, two of the tests turned up positive, both evidence of the spread of the cancer. There was a positive bone scan, and the chest x-ray indicated a "lesion" in my left lung.

By this time I was feeling betrayed by my breasts, so there was no problem in getting me to agree to the surgery—not even twice. When the surgeons suggested that when I recovered from this first surgery they would take the other breast, I was ready to hand both breasts over, although I was given no assurance that this would save my life, even with chemotherapy and radiation. This is because it is the nature of cancerous tumors to start shedding cells, which spread to distant parts of the body. So cutting off breasts at this point was akin to closing the barn doors after the horse has escaped. Adding chemotherapy and radiation added no promises, either.

The doctors (there were now three of them in the room) shook their heads in answer to my next question and said, "We don't know if you have three months, three years, or how long. We don't know if it has spread or, if it has, how far. We certainly don't know why; there's an awful lot we just don't know...."

Adding to my anxiety, I recalled that when I came in earlier that week, the doctor had looked at the plainly visible lump in my breast, and had asked with great concern in his voice, "Why did you wait so long to come in?" I went into instant panic and at the same time flew into a rage.

"What do you mean 'wait so long'?" I practically screamed. "I was just here three months ago and was told this... this...." I was sputtering by now. I calmed myself down, took a deep breath and said, "They told me this lump was only scar tissue from the previous biopsy." Six months before, I'd tried to tell them that this "scar tissue" was growing, but was repeatedly reassured that it was not and that everything was "normal." Three years before, I'd found the lump and was assured that it was "nothing to worry about."

"Never mind," he said, "We've got to schedule surgery right away."

I suddenly realized that the previous biopsy a year earlier had missed the cancer. Now it might be too late!

Having breast cancer was bad enough. To find out that the cancer had been growing in my breast for three years because of the inexperience, ignorance, or arrogance of a doctor was almost more than I could bear.

With eyes brimming with tears, I was experiencing the worst moment of my life. I wanted to scream, yell, hit out, rage, vent my fury, roll over, and die.

"Hey, wait a minute," I thought. "I'm not ready to roll over and die. I was fighting to live, and was going to fight this death sentence with everything I had. So, how could I afford to get angry at the very people I was counting on to help save my life?

If I had only a short time remaining, I needed to get busy. I had a lot of work to do. Thus began my Race for Life.

The Operation

Unfortunately, detaching me from my breasts wasn't that simple as it entailed fairly extensive surgery. But it wasn't that difficult, either. When I checked into the hospital for the mastectomy, the nurses who helped me unpack were amazed to see three complete sets of running clothes, three sweat bands, two pairs of running shoes, and not much else. I didn't bother with bras and regular clothing, feeling that I wasn't going to need them. I could see them shaking their heads as they walked out of the room. What they didn't understand is that I'd been a daily runner for fourteen years at that point and wasn't about to let this stay in hospital interrupt my routine any more than absolutely necessary.

On the morning of surgery, the head nurse walked into the hospital room to administer the pre-operative medication, the drugs routinely given to patients to allay anxiety and relax them. The bed, however, was empty.

"My God," the head nurse said to her aide. "She's run away! And we thought she was taking this so well." I'd been told the day before that the pre-op medication would be given to me at 5:00 a.m. I'd set my alarm for 4:00, crawled out of bed, slipped into my running clothes, tip-toed down the shadowy halls, and escaped into the still-dark hills surrounding the hospital. I covered six miles, enjoying one of the most satisfying runs ever.

All the fear, tension, stress, anxiety, and even the anger seemed to drain away and be replaced by a powerful feeling of being an Army general in charge of waging a war on a battlefield, my chest! The surgeons (four of them now!) were the colonels in charge of the operating room front; the nurses were in charge of the mop-up operations; and the rest of the medical support personnel, with their needles, tubes, and various areas of expertise, were awaiting their call to arms.

At the end of the sixth mile, I was ready to do battle. As I turned back to the hospital and approached the entrance, I was shocked to see my surgeon just arriving. He was even more shocked to see me! "What in the *world* are you doing here?" he asked incredulously. I actually felt a pang of guilt, because I felt sure that they'd never have given me permission to run if I'd asked.

As it turned out, the staff most certainly would not have allowed me to run. When you run, you sweat. Sweating causes dehydration. On the day of surgery, you can't eat or drink anything from the previous midnight on, so you tend to be a little dehydrated anyway. So, here was a sweaty, thirsty, and dehydrated patient "presenting," as they say, to surgery. The head nurse was chewed out for not keeping a closer eye on her charge, and the surgeon told the anesthesiologist to pump some extra intravenous fluids into me to compensate for the dehydration. The problem, however, was they had trouble getting the IV started because of my dehydration. It took three people and many "sticks" before getting into a vein. The surgeon walked in, saying, "Would you believe that this lady was out *running* this morning?" Under the influence of the numbing pre-op medications, I muttered, "See! No problem with running the day of surgery...."

The surgery went very well. I was wheeled from the operating room to the recovery room. As I was coming out of the anesthesia, I was already thinking about starting the exercises that the American Cancer Society's Reach to Recovery support group recommends. Because I was still pretty numb, I felt no pain and was raring to go. As I was trying to lift my arms, the surgeon walked in.

"What are you trying to do?" he asked, looking perplexed.

"I've got to get started on my exercises!" I told him.

He patted me on the shoulder and said gently, "I think we can wait a couple of days."

"Oh, okay," I said, and immediately fell back to sleep.

The next time I awoke, I *couldn't* move my arm. Each time I tried, there were sharp, stabbing pains. For a while, I tried just to "gut" through the increasing pain, but then I had this fuzzy series of thoughts: this is only temporary; there's no point in suffering like this; I might as well be comfortable; that's what pain medication is for. Finally, I succumbed to the siren call of the medication and slept.

The next day I was feeling a lot better and began to wonder when I could run next. When the doctor came by to check on me that morning, I asked him.

"As soon as you feel like it," he said.

"Well," I replied. "*When* do you think I'll feel like it?"

He chuckled and said, "Oh, knowing you, probably in a couple of weeks." He beamed as though he thought that was just *wonderful* news.

"A couple of weeks?" I replied. I was expecting him to say a couple of days! I was thinking of all the conditioning I'd lose by not being able to run for two whole weeks.

After he left, I got out of bed and started walking up and down the halls, pushing an IV stand, and prepared my body for a possible run the next day. That night I awoke a number of times, the pain still intruding on my sleep. My body required more medication and more time. The second day after surgery I was still a little weak and shaky on my feet. Disappointed, I thought, "Will I ever get back to running again?" It had been two whole days but it seemed like a month. On the third day, however, I felt great. "Today's the day!" I announced.

I think the poor nurses were in awe of this running-obsessed patient and yet they were totally supportive. I asked for a wide bandage to wrap around my chest. They brought me a twelve-inch wide Ace wrap which they then helped me swaddle myself with so that nothing could move—not that there was much left to bounce. But when the bandages were snug around me I found I could move with a lot less pain.

Triumphantly, I walked out of the hospital and broke into a tentative, gingerly jog. It felt wonderful! Tears came again to my eyes. But this time they were tears of joy.

A Race for Life

This book is the story of how I decided to turn my life around through a combination of three things: diet, extensive fitness training, and a can-do attitude. All three, I believe, have been vital in making sure that nearly twenty years after my operation, I not only have not had any further recurrence of the cancer, but am fitter, healthier, and happier than I have ever been.

In this book I talk about how important a plant-based diet is in creating optimal health and providing the right nutrients for strength and fitness. I also offer my experience of taking part in some of the toughest races in the world, and how I have found great companionship, personal fulfillment, and life-altering challenges in them. Thirdly, I provide practical insights into training your body and creating a positive attitude to all of life's challenges.

If all this seems a little overwhelming, then I don't blame you. It was overwhelming for me too at first. But I deeply believe that I am no more special or committed a person than anyone else. Like you, I have had moments of fear and doubt when I have not known where to turn. But I also believe that we all have the resources in our minds and our bodies that make no challenge insuperable and can provide us with a lasting sense of achievement. As I enter the second half of my seventh decade, I have neither felt better nor looked forward to life with more pleasure. I hope that my story inspires all of you—no matter how old you are or how physically challenged you may be—to stretch your capabilities and throw off the stereotypes of what someone your age or physical condition can do. If you are anything like me, you'll be amazed at what you can do! Moreover, if you follow some of the plans and ideas in this book, you'll get results. Why don't you join me in the race for life? I guarantee you will see results.

Chapter One

Enter the Diet, Enter the Exercise

If there is a cornerstone to my health, fitness, disease prevention and treatment program, it would have to be nutrition. After all, never did my very positive mental attitude, my belief that it could never happen to me, and my years of running prevent my developing cancer. Yet how I changed my diet happened by chance. Shortly after my diagnosis of cancer, I saw a tiny notice in a Honolulu newspaper that read:

Breast cancer and diet study being conducted. Those who have or have had breast cancer are invited to join a study to determine the benefit of diet in the treatment of cancer....

I couldn't believe my eyes. If the notice had read, "to determine the benefit of cosmic radiation in the treatment of cancer," I would have been on the phone in a flash. I had a feeling of total desperation. Only the slightest hint of salvation is enough to send cancer patients like me into orbit if that's what's promised. I can easily understand why "quack" cures are grasped at so desperately because that's how I felt. (You can read more about this in Chapter Three.) I'd also thought and been told that there was no way diet could have any influence on cancer. But here, at least, was hope!

I did not hesitate a moment. The advertisement told me to go to the office of Dr. John McDougall. When I got there, newspaper clipping in hand, Dr. McDougall explained to me why he thought diet was important to cancer. I learned that breast cancer rates in countries with a low-fat diet are low, while in countries such as the United States, where diets are high in fat, breast cancer rates are high.

So here was the answer to my question: "Why me?" I found out that the typical American diet consists of thirty-seven to forty-five percent fat, placing it among the fattiest in the world.[1] I also discovered that when women from countries with a low-fat diet migrated to countries with a high-fat diet, their breast cancer rates soon approximated those of their new country, if they adopted that country's diet. In other words, genetics did not seem to play a role in these incidents of cancer. Nor, so it seemed, did age. There was an increase in incidence of breast cancer in all age groups.

Even more important to me was the finding that when women in the low-fat diet countries got breast cancer, they lived much longer.[2] This fact really got my attention! Here was hope. Here was a chance to extend my life.

Was there any question about my changing my diet? None! Absolutely none!

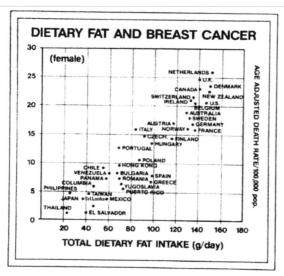

FIG. 1. *Breast cancer rates are highly correlated with the amount of fat consumed in the diet.*

No Chemotherapy and Radiation

There was a little "catch" though. Dr. McDougall advised me not to have chemotherapy and radiation. I was quite surprised, because I thought that in my case, considering the size of the tumor and the signs it had spread, it would be necessary. He explained that chemotherapy and radiation permanently damage the immune system and that I was going to need to have that system in excellent shape to stop my cancer reoccurring. He stated emphatically, "If you want to save your life, change your diet!"

I was confused. Whom should I believe? Which side should I go with? This was pretty scary now. There was one factor that made a big difference. Dr. McDougall pulled out the studies that supported what he was saying. The other doctors didn't.

I was now totally convinced. I changed my diet literally overnight and refused chemotherapy and radiation.

The Vegan Diet

The implementation of Dr. McDougall's meal plan was easy: If it was of plant origin, I ate it; if it was of animal origin, I didn't. This diet is called "vegan," but you needn't worry about terminology. I know you will have lots of questions: Aren't chicken and fish good for you? What about milk? What about protein and calcium? What about iron? What do vegans eat? Don't worry. All these questions will be answered in the course of the book.

Let me just say for now that the effects of my dietary change were immediate. In just twenty-one days, my blood cholesterol dropped from 236 mg/dl to 160 mg/dl. At the next test six months later it was 128 mg/dl. And the one after that was under 100! This practically eliminated my risk of heart attack, a result I hadn't even considered. When Dr. McDougall had seen my initial reading, he had told me I was at as great a risk of having a heart attack as I was of dying of the cancer. Here was another health shock because, as a marathoner, I thought I was immune to heart disease. (This was before one of the most famous of all runners, Jim Fixx, died of heart disease.)

I was shocked my cholesterol was so high, since I'd long before given up eating "red meat" and was a heavy exerciser. What I didn't know then is that chicken and fish have just as much cholesterol as beef and pork. I had not done my body any favors by switching the source of cholesterol.

It's not surprising that people think they're eating more healthily by choosing chicken and fish instead of beef and pork. The meat industries hide their cholesterol levels in chicken and fish through not mentioning them at all. Here, for instance, is an advertisement for beef that ran nationally in a popular magazine:

Cholesterol: perception vs. reality. This should make headlines: lean, trimmed beef has no more cholesterol than chicken—without the skin.

A fast-food chain advertised that: *Our mouth-watering ribs are as low in cholesterol as chicken and fish.*

The beef and pork industries must be hoping that their verbal manipulation gets past the public's awareness that cholesterol must be the same in all animals. "Low" means "high" in this case, about twenty-five milligrams of cholesterol per ounce of muscle—regardless of what animal it comes from.

We will discover more benefits of a vegan diet in later chapters.

Cholesterol Content (based on portion size)	
Food	**milligrams/100 grams**
Beef	70
Pork	70
Lamb	70
Chicken (skinned)	60
Turkey (skinned)	82
Halibut	50
Haddock	60
Tuna	63
Mackeral	93
Crab	100
Shrimp	150
Lobster	200
Cheese (Cheddar)	106
Liver	300
Egg	550
All plant foods	0

FIG. 2 Cholesterol content (based on portion size)

Enter the Exercise

A vegan diet was one aspect of my new health regimen. Training for the Ironman triathlon was another. (I will explain what the Ironman triathlon involved a little later.) As well as a lowered risk of stroke, colon cancer, and diabetes, one of the factors that most convinced me to become a vegan was that my race times started to improve. I was knocking off large chunks of time in every race I did. I concluded that my circulatory system had opened up, that my muscles were getting more oxygen and nutrients, and the waste products were being carried away faster. I could feel the benefits, and I knew that I was running, biking, and swimming a whole lot faster.

Other than the running that most children did, I had not been particularly athletic when I was younger. I ran my first road race in 1973. It was a three-miler, the Turkey Trot in Springfield, Ohio. It was small enough that I could start pretty close to the front. As I looked around, I could see nothing but men, and I smiled to myself, feeling pretty smug.

When the gun went off, I was nearly trampled. To avoid getting run over, I ran all out and almost died at the half-mile mark. My chest and lungs were screaming in agony, my legs turned to lead, and I felt as if I was dying. I had no choice but to slow down to nearly a walk. Slowly, I recovered enough to get back up to a halfway decent pace and hang on for the rest of the distance. I completed my first race and collected my very first trophy.

I would not forget those excruciating pains for a long time. My next race was over a year later, and although it was a four-miler, it was essentially a repeat of my first race. But again, I was rewarded with a handsome trophy (no other women, again). Having survived twice now, I entered a ten-kilometer (6.2 miles) race and noticed that the same sequence occurred no matter what the distance.

Races could be divided into a beginning, middle, and end. Beginnings were always great. All those horrible pains in my chest and legs signaled the end of the beginning. The middle began as I slowed my pace a little and the pains subsided. The end began as I saw the finish line and then it was trying to just hang on until I crossed it. In every race the sequence was the same—except in a longer race the middle began later and lasted longer.

It was another four years before I attempted a half-marathon. And guess what? It was exactly the same sequence! By then I'd had enough experience to realize that any distance I'd tried had the same ending: I crossed the finish line dying, with not much left. I did not realize then that this was the way it was supposed to be!

The leap from a half-marathon to a full one was a greater psychological battle. It was only when I was working in an all-male military office and saw these guys, many of whom were admittedly ten to twenty years younger than I, completing marathons with much less training, that I thought I could do the full marathon. I decided to break through those sex and age barriers. I just kept extending my long runs, gaining confidence along the way that I really could do it.

As I crossed the finish line at the end of my first marathon, I realized that I'd gone through the exact same sequence of beginning, middle, and end with nothing left.

Four years later I began to train for my first ultra-marathon (defined as any race longer than the standard marathon distance of 26.2 miles). Once my goal became an "ultra," the marathon seemed almost easy. That was an exciting discovery because I knew then that I could set any goal, and anything less than that was do-able, almost easy.

Running the World

Have you ever watched the amount of activity in a colony of ants? Do you notice how purposeful the ants seem to be? Each member of the group seems to know where he's going, what to do, and when to do it. These ants' entire lives are wrapped up in accomplishing genetically programmed goals.

Now look at humans. Some people seem to know what to do, how to do it, and when to do it. I never felt that fortunate. It seemed as though I was always looking at a whole bunch of options, found myself wanting more than one, then looking back at the choices I'd made, and wishing I'd done something else.

With the diagnosis of cancer, all that got swept away. I saw the crystalline blue of the ocean and lush green of the trees as if for the first time. Suddenly, just being alive was the essence of my life, and everything else was secondary. Then came a new and exhilarating sense of reckless abandonment and exciting opportunities.

I looked back at my life and saw where I was one of those ants just following the trail of the ant in front of me. I'd not dared to strike out on a trail of my own making. Cancer did for me what I was unable to do on my own. It plucked me from this trail of conventionality and dropped me in another place, one that seemed unique. Yes, other people had been diagnosed with cancer, but it seemed to me that they were in a different situation. My first two years after the diagnosis were spent assessing the illness and, after it appeared that I was not going to die immediately, I was free to plan the rest of my life.

Running has taken me all over the world. It is an exciting way to see new countries and meet people of different cultures who share a love of running. Planning a trip to China the year following my cancer diagnosis, I created and realized a fantastic dream: I ran the Great Wall of China. Well, not the whole length, because so much of it is in a state of disrepair. But I ran enough of it to get to experience the feeling of doing something so close to impossibility when compared to my old frame of reference.

Running along that magnificent, ancient creation was a joy in itself, but watching all the Chinese people watching me was the real thrill. Most of them had never seen a tall, fair, Western woman in a running singlet and shorts, and they must have thought I was crazy. After all, why would anyone want to run when they didn't have to?

Waves of drop-jawed Chinese parted and gawked in awe as I threaded my way through the crowds. They pointed at me, and then smiles played around their eyes. Then their lips widened, and their whole faces beamed. One elderly gentleman playfully ran alongside me, laughing uproariously. He was saying something in Chinese, and I was talking back in English. We communicated soul to soul perfectly, and I know we enriched each other's lives for a precious few moments.

After my return from China, I decided I wanted to backpack across Haleakala, the 10,000-foot volcano on the island of Maui known as the "House of the Sun." I scampered down the shale of the inside of the crater of the extinct volcano, hoping the vulcanologists were right in their assessment that it really was extinct. I peered down seemingly bottomless crevasses, saw two spectacular sunrises, and ran up the far side of the crater in a quarter of the time usually allotted for people to climb out.

As in China, I felt that this was really living, and wondered why I had waited so long to start! I had not yet even conceived of doing the "Run to the Sun." The following year I did it: running the 36.6 miles from the bottom to the top of Haleakala, completing it in seven hours forty-seven minutes and winning an age-group first place.

I have continually set myself new challenges. The fourth year after the cancer diagnosis (1986), I ran fifty-one races and placed in almost every one of them: thirty-three first places; nine second places; three thirds; and six races that were "fun runs" with no times or awards. These races ranged from a one-mile all-out sprint to three Ironman triathlons, and included numerous course, state, and international age-group records in running, biking, swimming, and triathlons.

In 1987, the fifth year after my cancer diagnosis, I did fifty-two races, again ranging in distances from the mile to the Ironman, with even more first place awards. In 1988, I changed my focus a little and ran the Moscow Marathon plus races in Kiev, Kharkof, Sochi, and St. Petersburg. Our interpreter there told all the Russians we met about me, this fifty-three-year-old "cancer patient" who does Ironman triathlons. I will never forget the looks of amazement on their faces. They wanted to know everything about my diet, training schedule, and how I got myself to do all these things. I delighted in the opportunity to talk to these people about the importance of diet, exercise, and a healthy lifestyle.

The Moscow Marathon was one of the more exotic marathons, and it was certainly one of the most memorable. This was before the Berlin Wall came down, when there were still animosities between the Communist countries and the West. What I found in running through the streets of Moscow was that the Soviets were intensely curious about Americans. They were extremely friendly and usually knew enough English to carry on a limited conversation. I spent so much time talking to foreign runners during that marathon that I had a terribly slow time, a P.W. (Personal Worst). But do you think that mattered? Being able to communicate with hundreds of people with immensely different backgrounds was hugely rewarding for me.

Since I wanted to take the "Aloha" spirit to the USSR, I carried, as part of my baggage, 5,000 Hawaiian orchids, which were distributed to the spectators along the course. The expressions of surprise and delight on the faces of the Russians were wonderful to behold. Even more wonderful were the soldiers from the Russian Army who'd been recruited to serve as course marshals along the 26.2-mile route. They stood at rigid, stone-faced attention. It was pretty exciting to see the stern, cold faces melt into smiles and big eyes as they realized what I was handing them. Being from Hawaii, I wanted to tell them how far I'd come to run in their marathon. That was when I discovered that they did not understand the word, "Hawaii." They'd just look at me totally puzzled, because there is no "h" sound in their language. When I found out that the Russian pronunciation for "Hawaii" was "G-vai," they all of a sudden understood, nodding their heads, eyes dancing, and big smiles on their faces. Ah, the importance of communication!

In 1989 I spent three weeks in Thailand and Nepal, doing every race I could find. Again, it was a similar experience. There were many opportunities to mix with the people, share my experiences, and tell my "story." People there could hardly believe that anyone would exert any effort that wasn't really necessary for survival. The concept of "exercise" is hardly necessary when you're at heavy labor all day long every day.

This was especially true in Nepal where people are so poverty-stricken that it seems almost criminal to waste any of the body's energy. What I saw was that food there was such a limited commodity and life so hard that there was no need to exercise or even have any choice in what to eat. The Nepalese already had an extremely low-fat diet and they "exercised" all day long and half the night—seven days a week, at that.

I also saw stress levels that were extremely high. I mentally compared their types of stress with the stress that we in America face with our deadlines, traffic congestion, noise, etc. These people worked long, hard days with no "coffee breaks" and rarely any days off. Even with all this heavy labor, some were not even making a subsistence-level living. Many could hardly feed their children, much less themselves. I can't imagine any greater stressor than seeing your children go hungry.

Ironically, the Nepalese, on average, were very healthy and lived to ripe, old, active ages. Obesity didn't exist. Neither did heart disease, nor most forms of cancer, ulcers, diabetes, osteoporosis, high blood pressure (hypertension), and arthritis. There went the theories that ulcers and high blood pressure are caused by stress, that lack of dairy products causes osteoporosis, and that arthritis is caused by "wear-and-tear." (See later chapters for more on these subjects.) As a result of the very positive changes in the way I felt and looked, I came to believe that diet plays an extremely important role in survival, health, and sports competition at any age. I think diet was at least partially responsible for shooting me into the international sports arena.

Extra! Extra! Read all about it!

My picture on the front page of the New Zealand *Herald* the day after my first place in the Ironman attests to the excitement felt by others. The headline across the top read, "Ruth, A Woman of Iron!" There was a similar reaction in Japan, Russia, Thailand, and Nepal. The headline in the *Asahi Shimbun* read, "American Woman, 54, Conquers Cancer, Conquers Ironman."

My races continued to increase year after year with my feeling stronger and faster. I have now won over 700 trophies and medals. I was even invited to the world-famous Cooper Clinic in Dallas, Texas to try and set a new age-group fitness record. This entailed getting on a treadmill that started out slowly and increased in both speed and incline, following a standard protocol. When you reached exhaustion, as everyone will sooner or later since the machine always wins, your time was noted and compared to others in your age group. This was a fantastic opportunity for me to demonstrate the importance of both diet and exercise to fitness. I first broke the fifty-five to fifty-nine group record in 1990, broke my own record the following year, and went back when I turned sixty and broke that record. It almost makes one anxious to get older. (Well, not really, but at least there are some rewards!)

In May 1998, *Living Fit* magazine sponsored a contest, seeking the "Ten Fittest Women of 1999." When a friend suggested I enter, I thought I wouldn't have a chance because I was so much older than the models seen in most fitness magazines. But, because of my long-term commitment to daily exercise, I felt I might have a chance and also wanted to prove that age does not necessarily deter fitness. Needless to say, I was pretty excited when notified, first by phone, and then by official express delivery letter, that I was one of the ten.

At last, as a "mature" woman (I no longer consider myself old, by the way) I feel as though I've come into my own. No longer could I consider myself an ancient relic to be put on the shelf or in a rocking chair, but one to be reckoned with in the sports world. Who'd have dreamed that anyone could go from that devastating cancer diagnosis to world champion triathlete and one of the fittest women in the world?

But what is the Ironman? And how did I get involved in it?

Chapter Two

The Ironman Itself

On October 11, 1986 I was sitting in the Honolulu International Airport, awaiting a flight to take me to Kona for my fifth Ironman Triathlon. I marveled that I was even there. Only seven months before I had been on my way to do an Ironman in New Zealand. When I won an age-group first place, I thought I was on top of the athletic world. That was in March, only five months after I'd done the 1985 Kona Ironman. If I were to do Kona again in 1986, that would have meant three Ironman triathlons in less than twelve months. I chose to give up doing Kona again and do New Zealand, figuring there was no way I could do both.

After the New Zealand Ironman, when someone had asked me what I was going to do next, I had wondered if I could do two Ironman triathlons in one year. (Conventional wisdom had it that the demands of an Ironman on the body are so great that a person can only do one a year.) Then in August I'd made another choice. It was either the Japan Ironman then or the Kona Ironman in October. I never even remotely considered the possibility of doing them both, of adding another Ironman triathlon in that same year although I was still doing running, cycling, and swim races every weekend.

Since I'd never been to Japan, and Continental Airlines had offered to sponsor me, I chose Japan. I fully expected to have to lower my goals as far as my performance was concerned but, to my surprise, I did very well and again placed first in my age group. That's when it occurred to me that my body might not be able to tell the difference between racing and training. At this point, however, I still wasn't sure. As long as I gave my body adequate rest time and the right fuel, maybe I could keep racing as frequently as I wanted to.

It never occurred to me I could do all three Ironman triathlons in the same year! In fact, I was sure I couldn't. People, especially my coaches, were always telling me I was racing too much. Since both the New Zealand and the Japan Ironman had gone so well, I decided to test the limits and do Kona as well. My heart started to race as I realized that, all my life, I'd set mental and physical limits for myself. And besides, if I had to drop out and not finish, what were they going to do: fire me?

Who'd have thought that a now-fifty-one-year-old "cancer patient" could do four Ironman triathlons in less than one year.

The First Ironman

Back in 1982, still recovering from my cancer operation, I gave myself a treat and visited my parents on the Big Island of Hawaii. My visit was timed, coincidentally, with the running of the 1982 Kona Ironman Triathlon. Standing on the sidelines of this grueling event, I watched awestruck as finishers completed the 2.4-mile swim, the 112-mile bike ride, and the 26.2-mile marathon. My brain had trouble handling what it was seeing. One side of my brain went, "This is humanly impossible! No one can do this much! It can't be done!"

"Yes, it can!" replied the other side.

"No, it can't! It's impossible."

"No, it isn't. Look!"

"No, no, nope, no way!"

For hours this went on as the finishers struggled across the finish line.

I'd already run several marathons and knew how I felt upon crossing that finish line—totally spent, exhausted, with absolutely nothing left! How could these people run a full marathon after having done a bike race which took the average competitor six to eight hours in extreme heat and after a swim which took from one to over two hours? It hit me with an intensity I couldn't believe.

As I continued to watch, an idea formed in my head. This time it was, "Maybe I could do that." Again I split into two voices.

"No, I couldn't possibly."

"Maybe I can."

"Forget it, that's crazy."

"Maybe if I trained hard enough."

"No way, impossible! Besides, you're too old." (Aged forty-seven seemed absolutely ancient to me at the time.)

"Well, maybe I could just try it...."

"My gawd, lady, even if you weren't too old, you're forgetting you're now a cancer patient!"

And that's where it ended...and began. An image of myself crossing that finish line was constantly in my mind. During my daily runs, I pictured that scene in Kona, Hawaii: the large finish-line clock, the tropical flowers surrounding the finish area, and the cheering crowds.

Yet I still wasn't sure. I told myself that there had to be a limit as to what I was physically able to do, and I did not want to set myself up for probable failure by reaching out for something that was totally unreasonable. And surely, for a middle-aged "cancer patient," this quest seemed totally ridiculous. This was "validated" by the fact that, as of that moment, no woman that old had completed the Ironman. Remember: we're talking about a 2.4-mile swim, a 112-mile bike race, followed by a full 26.2-mile marathon. I told myself that it would be absolute lunacy to even contemplate such madness.

During my regular, daily runs, my mind would wander. Images of my getting stronger kept coming up, and from time to time the thought of doing the Ironman would reappear. I started biking daily and right away began to push the limits of the rides, both in distance and intensity. I signed up for a master's (adult) swim class. I never really knew if I could do it and wished I possessed that "positive attitude" that everybody kept referring to. Then came the inspiration.

What if I, as a "cancer patient," could be the first to complete the Ironman Triathlon? The contrasting concepts—"cancer" and "Ironman"—intrigued me. Wouldn't that prove to myself that I really was a survivor and had beaten the disease? What if I took that damning diagnosis of cancer and turned it into the challenge of a lifetime and became an "Ironman" in the process? What if extreme super fitness could help fight cancer? What if getting my body the fittest it had ever been in my whole life was the best offense against the cancer cells that surely remained in my body? It was an exciting goal, something to wrap my life around, something worthy of a major commitment, for it would take a large part of my life.

I knew I was "falling in love" with a life with the Ironman. I started getting very serious about all three sports and even added weight training. I subscribed to magazines on all four, poring over them cover to cover. I looked for anything written on the triathlon I could find, not that there was much in those early days of the event. I started examining training schedules of every athlete I ran into. My obsession was total.

Then I noticed the physical and mental changes. My muscles became more defined, and it seemed new ones popped up all over. A friend, Bonnie K., one day looked down at me in mock disgust and shook her head, "You and your 'thirty-year-old' legs!" I slept like a rock and awakened after only five or six hours of sleep, raring to go for my morning run, quitting only because I'd run out of time. I ate like a horse and never gained a pound. I felt strong, confident, and, as if for the first time, I was really enjoying life. I'd found a challenge that was totally engrossing and could even forget about the cancer for short periods of time. More importantly, I also felt that I was on to something in dealing with the cancer.

What if there really never would be a "cure"? What if strengthening the body's immune system was the only way to deal with the cancer? I'd asked my oncologist how to build up my immune system to help fight the cancer. Shaking his head, he replied, "We don't know."

I developed a theory, and it revolved around both diet and exercise—to an extreme, although I now know that it's not as extreme as I'd originally thought. I also found it ironic that diet-oriented physicians disagreed with my exercise approach, and exercise-oriented physicians disagreed with the diet approach. Nobody, as far as I knew, had ever put the two together. It was scary, wading into these uncharted waters. But, after all, I felt I had little to lose.

Our bodies crave movement and when given time to adapt, can accomplish prodigious feats. This was true for even a by-now fifty-year-old body that I'd thought a few years earlier was already old! I was feeling younger—and certainly did not fit the stereotype of how a fifty-year-old woman would look and act. I also discovered that there are no limits—only those we set in our own minds.

That philosophy worked as I graduated from the Tinman triathlon (which is approximately a quarter Ironman) to a half-Ironman, and from a half-Ironman to a full one. In training for my first Tinman, I knew so little about training for cycling that I thought if I could just go the distance once, that was all there was to it. It was only after my first opportunity to go "all out" on the bicycle that I realized one had to go through the exact same sequence.

This entailed a start, with its accompanying chest and leg pains; the middle, with its backing off enough so I could stand the pain; and the end where the finish line was in sight. That was a major discovery for me, as I suspect it was for most others who were just venturing into triathlons in the early days where there were no "experts" to turn to and no texts to consult.

Then there was the matter of increasing the distances. In Hawaii, where I live, the shortest triathlon bike leg at that time was twenty-five miles. In 1983, the first half-Ironman distance triathlon in Hawaii took place and was known as the Windward Triathlon. I looked at that fifty-mile bike leg and wondered how I could possibly go that far. I did it, and then, of course, looked at a 100-mile bike leg and was again totally awed by that distance. Then the fifty-miler became "a piece of cake." I have not yet done a Double Century, a 200-miler, but I know that once I set that as a goal, the 100-miler should be easier by comparison, the secret to making "hard" seem "easy."

In later chapters, I will show you how to train for the three legs of the Ironman—running, swimming, and biking—although you don't have to run out and do an Ironman to get the benefit from exercise. Just know that I believe that you can do it if you really want to. Even if you don't want to run, bike, or swim, there are other exercises that provide benefits. Try jumping rope, climbing stairs, and even dancing! It all helps.

Chapter Three

Getting Informed

Triathletes are among the most sociable people I have ever met. I recall during the early days of running, cycling, and swimming, that my questions concerning the three sports were invariably answered totally, completely, and enthusiastically. The sharing of information seemed to be done so joyfully, and I found that I, too, as I learned the tricks of the trade, felt compelled to share with others.

First, I would respond to people who asked for help. Next, I started volunteering to share information—as in "Guess what I just found out!" Now, I share my knowledge in the form of seminars, talk radio shows, books, and videos with the hope of reaching people who never dreamt they ever wanted to know all about the joys of exercise, or running, swimming, and cycling!

As I watched and participated in the sharing of information, experience, and advice, I noticed that there was, unfortunately, from time to time, misinformation that was passed on. Indeed, I had even been a victim of some of these "fads," and it took me a long time to sort out fact from fancy. It's a process, by the way, that is far from ended, as the sport progresses and new equipment, techniques, and strategies are developed and become available to the people training and competing.

Consider this method for keeping elephants out of your back yard. All you have to do is, at exactly 6:00 every evening, sprinkle some pure water over the back gate.

"But," says a friend, "you don't have any elephants in your back yard!"

"See? It works!"

This is an example of superstitious behavior that sustains itself because it never fails to "work." This kind of rationale goes on all around you. See if you can spot some real-life examples of elephant repellents.

In the early days of my cancer diagnosis, a number of people would approach me with possible "cures." Some of them were so far out that I didn't even consider them. I did wonder, however, why so many others did. There were even glowing testimonies about their success rates.

How "Snake Oil" Cures Work

If you take any large group of patients with a disease, you'll find that regardless of how serious it is, the course of the disease is not a straight line to inexorable death. There are good days and there are bad days. This is known as "the natural variability of disease."[1] If you were to give all of these patients a dose of "snake oil," or some such preparation, you'd catch some of them at the bottom of a series of bad days and starting back up. With the dose of snake oil having just been given, it is assumed that the snake oil made them "better." We all have a tendency to want to create cause-and-effect links even when there may be none. When this happens, you've got a group of believers!

Those who are in-between or are at the top of a series of good days just need to be told they need to keep on taking their doses of snake oil, that it takes time for it to work. You probably won't hear from most of these patients again, anyway, so your reputation is safe. For those who died, it was "obvious" that they didn't start their snake oil soon enough.

If a self-proclaimed "expert" were to look deeply into your eyes and give you a diagnosis of "toxins in your lymphatics," it would be rude of your body not to feel better, especially if you then spent a lot of money on the snake oil remedy to rid your body of these "toxins." Then when you returned for a follow-up visit a week later, this same "expert" would look deeply into your eyes and pronounce you cured!

I have also observed that when one focuses intently on pain, it frequently changes its nature, sometimes even disappearing. The tendency, again, is to assign a causal relationship to the event.

A useful way to look at the total universe of knowledge and how it relates to us is to think of four boxes. In the first box there is all we know that we know. In the second box there is all we don't know but know we don't know. In the third box is all we know but don't know we know. And, in the fourth box, all we don't know that we don't know. Most of us are pretty comfortable with operating in the first and second boxes. Much of what we do day-to-day is on automatic because of knowing what we know. We know that we know how to get to work, for example. We know that we don't know how to get to a street we've never heard of. Knowing what we don't know usually keeps us from getting in over our heads and out of trouble. We know that we need a map. All the information in the third box keeps us limited. We don't know what we are really capable of because we never think to test it and, preferably, use it. Examples might be untried leadership ability or entrepreneurial skills that are too scary to test.

The fourth box, however—where we don't know what we don't know—is where so much potential lies. There's where the Great Beyond lies, and where our Unconscious has never been able to grasp knowledge by itself. It's only when we open ourselves up to others more knowledgeable than we are that we can be taken to realms we didn't even know existed. This is where I was with respect to diet.

These realms are different for each one of us. It's like living in a forest, never even suspecting there are such things as deserts, mountains, oceans, and space beyond the forest. These forest-dwellers may never know what they don't know. Or, take fish, for example. They know a lot about water but they don't know they know! This is why there is so much potential in our mental capacities. If we can tap into the tremendous resource of our brain-power, who knows what we can accomplish?

Here's an example of a myth and "not knowing that I didn't know" but thought I "knew what I knew." As a child I was told to always wait an hour before going into the ocean to swim. This was, after all, "common sense," because you could get stomach cramps and drown. As I started my heavy swim training and had to swim hard for two to three hours at a time, I found I couldn't sustain that workout without eating first. Then I found out that other hard-core swimmers ate first, too. This told me that the eat-swim-drown belief was a myth, so I revised my "knowing what I know."

It has been more than forty years since I've taken my college level philosophy and deductive logic courses. During this time I realized that I could really use a lot of the information I'd gained in those courses that I'd labored through as a college student, taking courses primarily to fulfill graduation requirements. Information that previously seemed to have little application to everyday life suddenly was a necessity in sorting out valuable information from mere coincidence.

It was ten years later, in 1969, while working on my Masters degree and a Ph.D., that I was sweating through graduate level statistics and courses in research design. It was another ten years before I really realized the value of being able to evaluate facts, hypotheses, raw data, theories, conjecture, trial-and-error, bell-shaped curves, improbable events, and freak accidents.

What little remained in my head after passing these courses suddenly had applications I'd never dreamed of. It was like discovering a Swiss Army knife in my back pocket when I'd been limping along using my fingernails as a screwdriver and my teeth as pliers. I marveled at how smart those professors of old were!

I started to see cancer patients on bell-shaped curves and placed people in the middle or ends of human distribution. I started thinking in terms of sample sizes and sampling errors. So what did it really mean if a friend had taken the latest electrolyte replacer and got his fastest ever time? There was also another friend who'd taken the same potion and bonked (hit the wall) so badly he'd had to drop out of the race. So here was one athlete swearing by this product and another cursing it.

When I tried it, I couldn't tell any difference because of the countless variables that varied so wildly I didn't know what was going on. The night before one race, I'd gotten an excellent night's sleep but had not had time for my usual pre-race bowl of oatmeal. The next race I'd been up half the night stewing about a problem, had awakened feeling totally exhausted, but had had plenty of time for the usual oatmeal breakfast. I may have also not bothered to put my fancy twelve-spoke racing wheels on, or decided to wear a tri-suit instead of making clothing changes. As I contemplated the almost infinite number of variables, I realized how nearly impossible it was to truly "know" anything!

To really "know" something, I would have had to have two large groups of athletes, one a control group with nothing varying, and the other the experimental group with one, and only one, variable. This is the only way to identify the effect of a variable; otherwise, you don't know which cause had which effect.

Can you imagine taking a hundred athletes and, for example, ensuring that they all got eight hours of quality sleep, all had four ounces of oatmeal with apple juice, all wore the same clothing, all used identical equipment, and all had the same level of motivation to win, etc? Next, I would have to randomly assign each one to either the control group or the experimental group. Then I would have to put on a race where the water conditions were identical for each swimmer, the winds the same speed and direction for each cyclist, and "footstrikes" identical for each runner. Then I would have to look at the finish times of both groups and calculate the mean (arithmetic average) finish times of both groups, and then determine if the difference, if any, was statistically significant (meaning that it is unlikely that this was a chance variation).

If there was a difference between the two groups, I might be able to conclude that the electrolyte replacer was the variable that made the difference. But, to be sure, the test would have to be repeatable by others.

The Placebo and Halo Effects

Do we dare consider the "placebo" and "halo" effects? The fact that one of the top triathletes recommends a particular electrolyte replacer sets the stage for this common phenomenon of "getting what you expect to get" (placebo effect). Or, when an "expert" predicts an event, whatever happens is frequently interpreted in terms of the expectation (halo effect), primarily because experts in one area tend to be viewed as authorities in other areas.

The mind is so powerful that it's quite possible that if you're told this little pill will make you go faster, you will! You can't possibly eliminate the placebo or halo effects when you are trying different food, equipment, or psychological processes. Even if you, the subject, don't know whether or not there's an active ingredient in a pill, there's a possibility of bias if the person giving you the pill knows. This is why experiments aren't valid and reliable unless they are double-blind, meaning neither knows what's in the pill. Some people want so badly to believe something, that no amount of evidence to the contrary will shake their faith.

This is especially true in the area of beliefs about food. How do you account for the fact that three-quarters of the world's population is vegetarian and yet most Westerners believe that to be healthy one must have dairy products and meat? This is especially baffling when there is a great deal of scientific evidence that animal foods are responsible for more than seventy percent of deaths in Western civilization.[2] Nobody wants to die and yet we keep eating the very same foods that cause heart disease, cancer, stroke, diabetes, osteoporosis, arthritis, and on and on. After I changed my diet and saw firsthand the very positive result, I wondered what other beliefs I might have that are so firmly entrenched that I dare not question them.

What about the people who think if "x" quantity is good, then "2x" will be twice as good, and "3x" will be three times as good? If I ran my best race on forty miles a week of running, just think what could do with eighty miles a week, the logic goes. And there are people who, incredibly, run 120 miles a week or more. The problem comes when some of us try to increase our training mileage to these levels and are rewarded only with injury. To go back to the example of the electrolyte replacer, if our experimental group was significantly faster, we then need to look at the quantity they drank. Assume it was twenty-four ounces. What would have happened if they had drunk only ten ounces, or fifty-two ounces? Now you see that we'd have to run another experiment, holding all other variables the same again, and have one control group and three experimental groups. And, are fluid levels of ten, twenty-four, and fifty-two enough levels to give us the optimum level of fluids? What if twenty-four ounces is too little and fifty-two too much? What if performance level increases up to forty-four ounces and starts to decrease with greater input? Our experiment with three levels could show that twenty-four and fifty-two are the same, with our "scientists" concluding that performance does not improve over twenty-four ounces.

The Fallacy of the Truncated Scale

Another factor to be considered in assessing the value or truth of data is the range or number of "data points" on the scale. Does the scale go high enough, low enough, or miss the optimum in the middle? This problem was vividly demonstrated in the so-called Harvard Nurses Study of the diets of 89,494 women where one of the findings was that fat in the diet did not influence breast cancer rates.[3] The trouble with this conclusion was that all the subjects had a high-fat diet, so there was naturally no difference in the breast cancer rates! In the meantime, however, a lot of damage is being done as women, and some of their physicians, are told not to worry about fat in the diet causing breast cancer. If the data points had gone low enough, with the dietary fat down to ten percent for example, the results would have been very different.

The error was repeated in this study with regard to exercise as well. The finding was that the breast cancer rates were no different between the "heavy" and "light" exercisers, the error being that their definition of "heavy" was too light. This is another example of the data points not going far enough—the fallacy of the truncated scale. Recognizing the problem, though, the survey-takers at least concluded that women should exercise anyway.

In addition to this, there are many arguments for individual differences. Some people assume that we are all basically alike, and others assume that we are so different we can't learn anything from each other. The truth lies in between. Within a broad range, we humans are remarkably similar, and within a narrow range we are as individual as our fingerprints. As a result, when assessing the outcome of someone else's experimental results, we need to consider whether the results fall within the narrow or the broad range. It's the similarities that allow blood tests to tell us, for example, that our iron and cholesterol levels are normal, or allow surgeons to perform the same basic operation on all of us. After all, it's pretty rare for a surgeon to open us up and find a real surprise! Of course, there are differences, and that's why we need, most of all, to keep an open, inquisitive mind, and be very careful about drawing conclusions. Once having drawn a conclusion, it needs to be held in the light of advancing knowledge. Know that when you find you are wrong about something, you are on the way to being right.

The essential thing to understand here is that you should get yourself informed about your health, but be sceptical about graphs and charts. My fitness plan, however, involves listening to your body, challenging what you can do, not depriving yourself of food or energy, and enjoying life.

Chapter Four

Changing Your Attitude

Have you ever had the experience of making a resolu-tion to make a major change in your life and then found your willpower crumbling in the face of a lack of support from the people and environment around you? One of the reasons that formal education is sometimes ineffective is that, although we can change behavior under classroom conditions, as soon as we go back to the old environment, the same old behavior appears.

One of the most basic tenets of learning theory is that behavior will recur if it is reinforced; and that which is not reinforced will be extinguished or drop away. Many people make resolutions to start an exercise program or resolve to start eating better and then find themselves back in the same old habits of not exercising or eating the same old foods.

What? Me Change?

Changing behavior can be considered a three-step process. First, you have to learn the theory. Secondly, the changed behavior must be elicited. Thirdly, it must be positively reinforced, or rewarded. All this means is that we need to know what to do, do it, and then want to keep doing it. With this powerful sequence, we can control our behavior and make ourselves do anything.

Since this book is about wellness, fitness, and overcoming disease, let's limit our discussion of behavior change to diet and exercise.

In my particular case, I was highly motivated to make a dietary change. After all, as I perceived the situation, the penalty for failure was death. My eating habits changed literally overnight. What then amazed me was that I started enjoying food more.

The most basic foods such as brown rice, apples, potatoes, broccoli, carrots, and oatmeal seemed, as if for the first time, to taste so good. I didn't need sauces, spices, sweeteners, etc., to make those foods appetizing. They were already delicious, and I started to appreciate their basic good tastes as if for the first time.

I had learned the theory: that a low-fat diet seemed to enable people to live longer. I was highly motivated to adopt it. Then the reinforcement was the rediscovery of the good taste of pure, healthful food and feeling better.

You're the One Who's Sick, Not Me!

The only difficulty lay in my environment. My then husband apparently did not see any value for him in eating this way, saying, "You're the one who's sick, not me!" I was even accused of becoming "a religious zealot" in terms of the enthusiasm with which I embraced the dietary change.

Had I not had the negative motivator of fear behind me, I'm not sure that I could have stuck with the change. After all, I could not clear the kitchen of all the offending foods and had to face the challenge of continuing temptation. I must say, though, that after learning about the problems that meat and dairy products cause, I was not all that tempted.

It was a little different with friends in a social environment. Those who knew of my change were afraid to eat in front of me and thought that I would never find anything to eat at restaurants. Things have changed a lot since I became a vegetarian. Not only are almost all restaurants happy to prepare a vegetarian meal, but there are lots of vegetarian options for you to try.

Ethnic restaurants are probably a fairly safe bet, because the menus offer dishes from generations of people who obviously survived on that diet. Mexican restaurants are great because you can order side dishes of rice, beans, and corn tortillas. (Note: you may have a choice between corn and wheat tortillas.

Wheat tortillas are usually made with refined, white flour, so go with the corn tortillas.) This makes an absolutely scrumptious meal and you'll be amazed at how inexpensively you can eat, too! Chinese and Japanese restaurants already serve fairly healthy dishes. Just go for the soba (buckwheat) noodles and vegetables. More and more restaurants are now serving brown rice. I always ask for it even if I know they don't serve it. I want them to know that the demand is there. You can also ask them to prepare the food with no added oils, or to skip the monosodium glutamate (MSG) if you're on a low-sodium diet. Again, these meals are usually delicious as well as inexpensive. Indian restaurants are also good bets for healthful eating. Many of them have a great selection of vegetarian dishes such as curries, dal, and chapattis. I have included some recipes at the back of this book for you to make at home.

Groups are Powerful Stuff

With regard to making exercise changes, we already know in theory that exercise is good for us and most of us never get enough. How do we put into practice resolutions to exercise more and get to the reinforcement?

One secret I've found is to join a group. This has been powerful motivator for me. First, a group usually has a leader or coach who provides instruction and encouragement. Secondly, peer pressure can do wonders in terms of making us want to keep to a task and do it well. The social aspects of groups satisfy other needs as well, such as companionship, role models, like-minded friends, and in some cases compatible lovers.

For about fifteen years I was a solitary runner. I ran the same course, the same distance, used the same running style, and did not improve much. Once I joined a formal group of runners headed by the legendary New Zealand ultra-marathoner, Max Telford, my progress was exciting. I was increasing my distance easily because of the fast friendships that enabled me to run miles painlessly while talking and having lots of fun. We tackled steep hills, bounding and striding up them, laughing all the way. At the end of our workouts, we basked in the good feelings we all had for our training efforts and each other. At races we sought each other out and reinforced each other's efforts.

As I got more into road races, I started to work out on a regular track. Here I was, at the age of forty-seven, learning a whole new vocabulary consisting of "400's," "800's," "intervals," "quarters," and finding out that running around in circles could actually be fun. This group still trains every Wednesday evening at the University of Hawaii under the tutelage of the women's track coach, Johnny Faerber.

I miss a workout only under the direst of emergencies. To illustrate, I recall once getting off a plane after a five-hour flight from Los Angeles to Honolulu and going directly to the track to run! I've done 100-mile around-the-island bicycle rides, gotten off the bike, and done a track workout. This is in spite of occasionally being so saddle-sore that I could barely walk.

Swim training in a pool can be so boring that I can hardly ever bring myself to do it alone. Yet, with a group it is actually fun. Coaches are a necessity here, because swim technique is critical to racing fast, and swim form deteriorates rapidly under fatigue. Even when not tired, it seems that I need constant reminders to keep my elbows high!

The bike rides I mentioned above would never have been undertaken alone. In the first place, I always do long rides using the buddy system. It's the safest thing to do in case of accident or mechanical failure. Secondly, a boring ride is transformed into something joyous when riding with compatible people. The experiences we share are so reinforcing that I'm hooked even when not training. And it must work for others as well since we always have a nice, large, and willing group.

As a fringe benefit we see some of the most glorious sights in the world. In Hawaii, on the island of Oahu, we start out by climbing over Diamond Head, go past Hanauma Bay, scream downhill to Sandy Beach and see some of the most beautiful rocky seacoasts on the island. On clear mornings, you can see all the way to the outer islands of Molokai, Maui, and Lanai. These experiences are so exciting I wish I could share these with the whole world!

As you can probably tell, I'm something of a health evangelist! I try to get people out on the roads or in the ocean, just as I implore people to try eating a diet of 100 percent plant foods for just twenty-one days. Many have said they'd try it, have loved it, and are still out there. A few have tried it, intended to get back to it, and somehow never quite made it, but still loved it. And some will not even try it. Those people in the first two groups are your athletic supporters, and people in the third group are your non-supporters. Surround yourself with athletic supporters, and you won't have any problem maintaining a healthy and fun exercise and diet program.

Chapter Five

Changing Your Diet

When I made the switch to a vegan (strict vegetarian), low-fat diet, I found that, for the first time in my life, my bowels functioned the way they were supposed to. In previous years I could not eat very much food for fear of gaining weight. I was, as a result, always hungry and had rabbit-pellet-sized stools which were brought forth only under great strain. I thought, because physicians had told me, that two or three bowel movements a week were probably "normal" for me. The day after I changed my diet I discovered what "normal" is supposed to be!

It is very obvious from all the TV, radio, magazine, and other ads that constipation and hemorrhoids are common in this country. Had I weighed and measured the stools of other cultures, as did Sir Denis Burkitt, M.D., I would have found out that most of these people had large, bulky, soft stools that moved effortlessly, frequently, and had a transit time (time of travel from mouth to anus) of eight hours or less as opposed to thirty-six to fifty-two hours seen in this country and England where Sir Denis did his ground-breaking research.[1] I would have also found out that there were entire societies without a single case of hemorrhoids—indeed, they did not even know what they were.

No longer was I plagued with having to worry about being able to move my bowels before a race or with having to make an emergency pit stop during a race. A proper diet actually normalizes the intestinal tract, and I have had to relearn this lesson occasionally, usually when I am traveling and not able to get my usual amount of fiber.

Diverticulosis is another affliction that is common in this country and rare in low-fat, high-fiber–diet countries. Diverticula are little "outpouchings" that occur in the intestines when the peristaltic (muscular contractions) movements do not have enough bulk to "grab." It's rather like inflating a balloon with weak spots. The weak spots in the intestines bulge out and create little pockets. These diverticula are prone to irritation, inflammation, and infection, and can be very painful. When the condition reaches this stage, it's called diverticulitis and, like so many other afflictions in this country, it's preventable.

Amazingly, another preventable side effect so many people in this country suffer from is hunger pangs. This is caused from not having enough food in the stomach. Many people try to control their weight by just eating less, the "push away from the table" method, and, therefore, suffer from hunger. The problem is that it doesn't work. Even if they manage to lose a few pounds, once they go back to their old ways of eating, they gain all the weight back, and then some. Compare the difference between 100 calories of oil (one tablespoon) and 100 calories of potato (a large one). Which will do a better job of filling you up?

Double or Even Triple Your Pleasure!

What most people don't know is that they can actually eat two to three times as much food (quantity-wise) and still lose weight! Most plant foods are very low in calories, so one can fill up and feel satisfied on this program. The exceptions are nuts, seeds, avocados, olives, and coconuts.

Since the hunger drive is one of the most powerful of drives, most people who try to deprive themselves soon succumb and will frequently go overboard once they decide "the heck with it" and the body compensates for the period of "starvation." Then come the guilt pangs, new resolutions, and the cycle begins again. Then, because the body senses that the starvation period is over with and food again is plentiful, it starts restoring (re-storing, literally) its fat reserves. It does this as a survival mechanism to get ready for the next period of "starvation." The bad news is that the body gets more efficient at laying in fat stores, and you end up with a higher body-fat percentage and a lower lean body mass. This means there is less muscle with which to burn up calories, and that is one reason why the body puts the fat back on more easily.

This is also why exercise is so important; it combats the tendency to lose muscle and may, in fact, add it instead. That is why low calorie diets don't work. Whenever you start restricting food intake, you are up against this most powerful of survival mechanisms. If people only knew that they could eat as much as they wanted, that they could eat until they were completely satisfied, and that they could even lose weight on such a plan, wouldn't you wonder why they wouldn't all do it? Boy, I sure do!

I have all my favorite foods, starting in the morning with oatmeal, bananas, and raisins moistened with water or apple juice and a teaspoon of blackstrap molasses. This is quite filling and sustains a good early morning workout or race. From then on, I usually "graze" on whole grains, vegetables eaten raw—such as carrots, broccoli, and cauliflower—and fruits like apples, oranges, and more bananas and raisins.

Lunches and dinners are usually centered on potatoes or rice. Sweet potatoes, yams, and regular white potatoes can be sliced and microwaved for five or ten minutes for nearly instant satisfaction. One of my favorite foods is plain brown rice. Its nutty, chewy flavor is so superior to white rice that I find it amazing that some people still eat the white. Besides tasting better, brown rice is much higher in fiber and the vitamin-B complex. I cook mine in an automatic rice cooker, using two-to-one proportions of water to rice. It doesn't even take any longer to cook, being usually ready in about twenty-five minutes. It's even faster in a pressure cooker. I love brown rice plain or as a base for chili, tomato-based sauce for Spanish Rice, or with water-sautéed chopped vegetables a quick and easy chop suey.

Dessert is usually a large (four-quart size) bowl of air-popped, plain popcorn. This keeps both hands and mouth fully occupied and has all kinds of positive benefits—such as lots of fiber and vitamin-B complex—and tastes great once you get past the need for salt and butter.

I have been eating like this for almost twenty years. What I've found is that plain, whole, unprocessed food can taste great. I'll admit that I made the dietary change literally under the threat of death. But I also immediately rediscovered the wholesome good taste of pure, plain, unadulterated food.

But What Does It Do for Energy?

I found my energy levels soaring! Wouldn't you agree that this would have to be the case in order to train for an event like the Ironman Triathlon? I rarely take a day off from training, and when I do it's usually from the press of other business. I rarely cut short a workout, and when I do it's most frequently from running out of time.

I sleep like the proverbial rock and rarely suffer from any kind of depression or moodiness. The most frequent comment I hear from my coaches and friends is that I race too much. I'm delighted when I hear this from "youngsters" twenty to thirty years younger than me. And, in fact, I do race a lot, as detailed in my first chapter. I've been doing on the average fifty races a year ever since my diagnosis, and hit a new high of sixty-three races in 1997. That is at least one race almost every weekend all year around. I would do more except that most of the races start at the same time, 7:00 a.m. Sunday mornings!

But Where Do You Get Your _____ (Fill in the Blank)?

I cite all this as evidence that a vegan, low-fat diet can't be all that deficient in calories, protein, calcium, essential fatty acids, minerals, and all those other factors that detractors usually quote.

Calories come from all the macronutrients—protein, fat, and carbohydrates. The preferred source of energy for our muscles, however, is carbohydrates. The best source of carbohydrates is plant foods; in fact, animal food provides little if any carbohydrates. Getting enough calories is a matter of balancing calorie-dense foods such as grains and dried fruit with low-calorie density foods such as green, leafy vegetables. This is how to control weight loss and weight gain.

There is no way that you can be deficient in protein as long as you are eating enough in calories. You will also get all the essential amino acids with a plant-based diet since all vegetables and grains contain adequate amounts of all the essential amino acids. Some people will have to go back and read that sentence again. In the popular press I have frequently found the perpetuation of the myth that either you need animal protein or you need to "combine" protein, or that soy beans are the only complete protein. None of this is true, and it becomes obvious when one looks up the essential amino acid content in foods such as rice, potatoes, corn, oats, broccoli, taro, and all the green, leafy vegetables. These foods possess complete proteins and if eaten in sufficient quantity to satisfy calorie needs will satisfy our protein needs.

The problem in Western society, however, is not one of getting enough protein; it is rather getting too much protein. And if that protein is of animal origin, you put yourself at risk for osteoporosis, kidney failure, arthritis, allergies, and respiratory problems such as asthma, mucous formation, and sinusitis.

You will get enough calcium since you are getting it from the same sources that cows, horses, elephants, and rhinos get theirs—which is plant foods, primarily greens. In any case, the problem is usually not one of calcium deficiency but of protein excess. When you eat too much protein (amino acids), the body has to buffer all that acid, which it does with calcium from our bones.

Fat

People frequently say, "But we need some fat in our diet." Yes, we do need some. These are the essential fatty acids, which we get from most every food we eat. For example, lettuce is thirteen percent fat, celery six percent fat, and oatmeal sixteen percent fat. The problem is not that we're getting too little fat but that we're usually getting too much.

This also means no added vegetable oil or margarine. You don't need it, and if you add it, it raises your dietary fat percentage to levels where cancer, especially breast cancer and probably prostate cancer, becomes a risk. Margarine is not a good substitute for butter for a number of reasons. Although margarine has no cholesterol itself, because it has to be hydrogenated to make it solid at room temperature, unnatural fat is created. In order to manufacture margarine, the fat molecules must be converted to trans-fatty acids, a key component of hardened vegetable oils. This formation of trans-fatty acids alters the structure of the fat molecule. Besides raising cholesterol, the use of margarine blocks the action of prostaglandins which help to lower blood pressure and increase removal of sodium from the body.[2] All fats—margarine and vegetable oils as well—seem to increase the incidence of all types of cancer. So, it seems not to matter whether it's saturated, monounsaturated, or polyunsaturated. Keep your fat percentage as low as possible. T. Colin Campbell in the China Diet Study found that the lower the fat, the healthier the people, down to five percent of calories from fat.[3]

Lots of people feel so much better eating this way that most who have switched would never go back to the old way. What I have found is that this eating program actually promotes an exercise program. You do more because you feel so good!

What about Carbo-loading?

Carbo-loading is a technique used by some athletes to increase the amount of glycogen, a carbohydrate in the form of sugar that the muscles can use. When you have a hard training bout or a race, you use up your glycogen. You then need to replace it by eating carbohydrates. If you are eating a vegan diet, you don't need to do anything different since you are carbo-loading every day. As a result, you are always ready for anything—training or races in most any sport!

The Secret to Health and Fitness

I remember one day after completing a two-mile swim having a "revelation": The "secret" to health and fitness is what you put in your body and how you move it around. The idea should be to put in nothing but good food and move it around with lots of exercise. It all seems so simple. Every one of the trillions of cells in our body has three requirements: nutrients, oxygen, and removal of waste products. The proper diet takes care of the first and exercise takes care of the second and third!

This chapter on nutrition would not be complete without addressing one of the most common plagues of the Western world—obesity. Obesity is actually a symptom of an improper diet in conjunction with a sedentary lifestyle. There are people who go from one diet to another, or one commercial weight loss program to another. They've spent literally thousands of dollars and still have fat, overweight bodies.

The issue with many people is cosmetic. This is best illustrated by the popularity of liposuction surgery. With these people, health is obviously not the major motivator—aesthetics or cosmetics are. This is not to put down the importance of feeling good about how you look. I think that looking good is extremely important and plays a major role in our self-esteem. You just need to know that you can have a beautiful, slim, sexy body by adopting the lifestyle that will give this to you.

Since the majority of this population will at some time in their life go on a calorie-reduction diet to try to lose weight, let's talk a little more about why weight-reduction or calorie-restricting diets don't work. As soon as you go off the diet and back to eating the diet that caused the problem in the first place, you'll likely regain all the lost weight and then some, because the body "learns" how to deposit fat more efficiently.

Okay, Limit Your Oxygen!

There's no way to beat the system. We humans have, for the most part, pretty strong survival mechanisms. For example, we need oxygen. Now, try to deprive yourself of air. True, you can hold your breath for a couple of minutes, but the drive to breathe will prevail. Try to deprive yourself of sleep. True, you can stay up one, two, or maybe even up to ten nights, but the drive to sleep will also prevail. After only a day or two, the brain will be grabbing micro-sleeps. Now, try to deprive someone of food. Tell them that they can eat only seventy-five percent of what they normally eat. They probably will start obsessing about hot fudge sundaes, chocolate candy bars, and banana splits. They probably could stick to the seventy-five percent program for a little while, depending on the rewards, but not for very long.

Can you imagine a weight loss center saying to you, "Okay, we're going to put you on a restricted oxygen diet. You can only take three-quarters of your normal breath for the next week. Check back in with us, and we'll see how you're doing"?

Since you're all motivated, you charge out the door determined to follow the instructions. How successful do you think you will be?

Well, you're dealing with a very similar situation when you tamper with the drive for food. "Willpower" will keep you going for a little while, but your drive for survival should win. If it doesn't, you risk ending up like Karen Carpenter, the popular young singer who died of anorexia. Even if your "willpower" lasts long enough to get your weight down, it will not stay down when you go back to your old eating habits. Most people will soon chuck the whole idea and binge to make up for the lost food. That's why the whole system of dieting fails, regardless of whether it's a self-imposed, medical, or commercial program. (You can read more about obesity and weight control in Chapter Eight.)

In order to lose weight and keep it lost, you must make a lifestyle change, and this lifestyle change must include a change to a low-fat diet along with lots of exercise. There's been a lot of press lately on best-selling books on dieting that proclaim that low-fat diets don't work. They promote high-protein diets instead. But these books are not telling the truth about those folks who are successfully living on a low-fat, vegan diet. The vegan diet does work, and there are millions who are here to attest to that fact.

The other part of the problem is that people want to hear that it's all right to eat the animal foods they think would be too difficult for them to give up. The sad news is that the health of these people is severely compromised in the long run. The answer is to let the body eat as much as it wants just as it breathes and sleeps as much as it wants. It will, anyway! None of this is in your control. What you can control, however, is what food is available.

A weight control program begins with your grocery shopping. My rule is to shop only at the edges of the store. Depending, of course, on the layout, you'll find the produce section on one end and the breads on another. So you can go "hog wild" with the vegetables, fruits, and whole grains.

If It Has a Face or a Label, Don't Eat It!

Here's a little rule of thumb: If it comes from anything that had a face, eyes that look back at you, or had a Mom and a Dad, don't eat it. If it fits those criteria, it also has muscles, and all muscles have cholesterol and saturated fat. These two substances cause major damage to our bodies, clog our circulatory system, and depress our immune system. Cholesterol leads to heart disease and strokes; saturated fat to cancer. These are the first, second, and third causes of death in this country. That's why I promote a vegan diet—no animal products whatsoever.

Another little rule I follow came about as a result of hearing all the admonitions to read the food labels. Labels are only found on foods that come in boxes, cans, tins, or jars. This rule is: If it has a label on it, don't eat it; or at least be very suspicious! Now I know that may sound a little extreme, but if it has a label, it usually means that it's been processed, i.e., had something removed or added. Either way, you lose.

Stick to whole foods and you can't go wrong. All one has to do is look at elephants, giraffes, and most primates and realize that they get all the nutrients they need from plant sources. These vegetarian animals, by the way, have a much longer life span than meat-eating animals do, living more than twice as long.

But You Do Eat Fish, Don't You?

I hear this question all the time, and then I see the shocked expression that follows my emphatic, "No, absolutely not!"

Predictably, the response is, "But what's wrong with fish?" Well, there's a lot that's wrong with fish.

We know that too much animal protein increases your risk of osteoporosis (see Chapter Six) and fish qualifies as a concentrated source of protein. Since most people get too much protein, we don't need fish for that reason. What about the omega-3 fatty acids that are supposed to be so good for you? Well, if you are eating a diet with lots of leafy green vegetables, you are getting your omega-3 fatty acids from the same source that fish do—fish get their greens from seaweed or algae.

The flesh of fish is also one of the most contaminated of foods. Even fish found in open oceans are exposed to pesticides, herbicides, and heavy metals such as mercury, lead, cadmium, and arsenic. They are also sources of hepatitis, polio, E. coli, *Salmonella, Ciguatera* poisoning, and an array of parasites such as *Anasakis simplex* (a gastrointestinal worm), and *Clonorchis sinensis* (a liver fluke).[4] So, there are many reasons to eat a plant-based diet and no reasons not to. Besides, this diet tastes delicious and makes you feel fabulous. What else could you ask for from a diet?

Getting Started: Food Tips and Recipes

Setting up your kitchen is much easier on this program. The following kitchen tools are useful: baking dishes, chopping block, cooking spoons, colander, grater, measuring cups and spoons, mixing bowls, muffin tins, paring and chopping knives, pizza pans, non-stick pots and pans in various sizes, soup ladle, sprouting jars and lids. I also cannot get along without my automatic rice cooker, slow-cooker, air-popcorn popper, and electric wok for an almost infinite variety of stir-fry (with water) dishes.

Staple foods to keep on hand are a variety of whole grains (oatmeal, brown rice, wheat berries, buckwheat flour, etc.), vegetables (potatoes, carrots, cabbage, onions, garlic, tomatoes, broccoli, etc.), fruit (bananas, apples, berries, melons, raisins, etc.), and spices (basil, chili powder, cumin, mustard, oregano, sage, thyme, turmeric, etc.). With these foods on hand, you can make a healthful variety of delicious meals.

The following are guidelines for beverages, meals, snacks, desserts, and cleanup. At the end of the book is a seven-day meal plan and supporting recipes.

Beverages: The best drink in the world is nature's purest: water. It used to be considered gauche to order water as your beverage in a restaurant. Thank goodness those days are long gone. Since I frequently have just come from a workout, I am usually very thirsty and not only order water but a very large glass of it. The same is true if I'm at a party, cocktail or otherwise. If I really want to celebrate, I'll have a club soda with a twist!

For variety's sake, there are two other beverages that I recommend. First thing in the morning, as a coffee substitute, mix one teaspoon of blackstrap molasses in a cup of hot water. Not only is this beverage stimulant-free, but it also gives you a good percentage of the day's allotment of iron, calcium, and other minerals.

The second beverage that I keep on hand in the refrigerator is a large jug of lemonade—the old-fashioned kind. I squeeze half a lemon into a half-gallon jug of water, adding just enough sweetener to take the edge off. This is a wonderful, healthy thirst-quencher. It is also the only juice I drink and I don't strain it. In general, I eat the whole fruit to get the entire fiber and the bulkiness that fruit gives. It helps keep the appetite under control, too.

Breakfast: My breakfast usually consists of a bowl of oatmeal, cooked very quickly in a microwave oven (two minutes) or sometimes not even cooked because I like it raw, too. It does not matter whether it's regular or quick cook-ing oatmeal since the quick cooking version is just rolled thinner. I add raisins, bananas, and a little blackstrap molasses to make a wonderful, filling treat. Then in order to boost its nutritional value, I add greens. This may sound a little strange to some of you, but just try it! The first time I tried this was when I was at the 1988 Seoul Olympics at the athletes' training table. Because there were so many Asians and many of them ate greens in the form of seaweed for breakfast, I decided to try it and liked it. Then I tried other greens such as kale, edible hibiscus, and even cabbage. Since greens are the "gold standard" of nutrition, I try to get them as often as possible, even at breakfast.

For special breakfasts, I make pancakes or waffles. For toppings, I add applesauce or fruit purée. Naturally, I skip the butter or margarine: It's not at all necessary for a satisfying taste once you get used to the delicious flavors of the other ingredients.

This selection also works for breakfasts eaten out. You can almost always find pancakes on the menu. Some of the more health-conscious restaurants make whole wheat or buckwheat pancakes, which, of course, are better for you than the standard white flour-mix pancakes. Again, be sure to leave out the butter and margarine. While others may be raising their cholesterol and fat levels with egg-based breakfasts, you can be doing your body a favor and enjoy your breakfast just as much.

Lunches: Mid-day meals can consist of any one of many different selections. Some possibilities are: baked or microwaved potatoes with carrot and broccoli sticks, whole wheat pita bread stuffed with sliced mixed vegetables, a whole wheat bagel with an orange and an apple, brown rice mixed with frozen succotash, and so on. This can also make a great brown-bag lunch.

One of my favorite ploys when I'm eating out and something like roast beef sandwiches are being served, is to ask for a "bread sandwich"! This also works in fast food places as well. A whole grain bun or a couple of slices of bread along with a salad (greens, tomato, bell pepper, onions, etc.) stuffed in between is adequate, especially if it's a rye or whole grain bread. Whole grain sourdough bread is also sometimes an option.

Dinners: My last meal of the day may be any one of the options listed above. If I feel like cooking, I make one of the following recipes:

- Spaghetti made with whole-wheat pasta and sauce made with tomato paste, onions, garlic, bell peppers, chopped broccoli, and seasonings, (the chopped broccoli flowerets can fool people into thinking you've got meatballs in the paste!).
- Chili made with kidney beans, tomato sauce, onions, garlic, bell pepper, chili powder, and lots of brown rice.
- Pizza made with a whole-wheat crust covered with a tomato-based sauce with chopped green onions, round onions, bell peppers, mushrooms, and alfalfa sprouts. For an "instant" crust, use pita bread or chapattis.

One of the nice things about eating this way is that you can modify almost any of your old favorite dishes. Just skip the animal products, fats, and oils.

When you skip meat, increase the veggies. When you skip oils, increase the water. If you need to stir-fry or sauté anything, do it with water or soy sauce. It works very well.

Go to some of the ethnic grocery stores to get ideas for some really interesting foods. For example, Asian grocery stores in your neighborhood sometimes sell many different types of rice. Salads are usually a healthy selection, but can be pretty dull if they consist of the usual iceberg lettuce with a slice of tomato. While browsing through the produce section, look at the variety of cabbages and other greens available, especially some of the newer varieties. They are usually inexpensive, especially relative to meat, and make such interesting combinations of dark greens, reds, and textures. You can also add snow peas, bean sprouts, corn, okra, eggplant, or whatever you see that looks good. Get creative with some of the gourmet greens now available!

With regard to salad dressings, I long ago decided to skip them. I love salads just plain. For those who can't handle that, sprinkle some Balsamic vinegar or lemon juice on the veggies.

Grazing: This is what I do between meals: I nibble on fruit, carrots, whole grain breads, air-popped popcorn, sweet potatoes, almost anything I have in the house. If you keep the high-fat foods out of the house, they can't tempt you. Remember: With this way of eating, you get to eat a lot, eat often, and not gain weight as long as you are exercising enough.

Desserts: To satisfy that sweet tooth and still have a healthy dessert, try any of the many varieties of fruits in season. Or, if that's not an option, frozen fruit is a possibility. I especially like air-popped popcorn and have it every night. I like it just plain, but if you need to flavor it, spritz it with diluted soy sauce or sprinkle cinnamon on it.

Cost: One last point concerns expense. You will be amazed how little this food program costs. Nobody believes me when I tell him or her how little I spend a month on food. I walk out with sacks of groceries because potatoes, cabbage, onions, papayas, apples, oranges, bananas etc. are very bulky, giving you a lot for your money.

One of the reasons you save so much money is that you are not paying for fancy packaging. This can be one of your contributions to the well being of the planet by not producing so much garbage. Remember there's no "away" when you "throw your garbage away." You will be doing your part in protecting the environment from the ravages of our industrial society, with its wanton use of resources to make all this packaging available. But, primarily, the cost is less because it requires no labor to process and refine natural foods. And there's less labor for you, too. It really doesn't take all that much time to prepare your own foods. You don't need a lot of fancy recipes to make good, nourishing, filling meals—unless you want to. I have written a cookbook with over 100 recipes that meet my CHEF criteria, Cheap, Healthy, Easy, and Fat-free.[5] These are recipes that I acquired or developed over the years that make fueling your body "a piece of cake." You can find some at the back of this book.

Oh, yes. There is another advantage that you will enjoy. Clean-up is so much easier and faster without grease splatters and with no oily film on dishes, pots, and pans, Even your sink drains will cheer! So how can you pass up such a deal? You can help yourself to glowing good health, save money, and be an environmentalist at the same time.

Chapter Six

Osteoporosis:
The Hidden Handicap

S itting here at my newly found friend, a not-too-user-friendly computer, I am building stronger bones. I am sipping my coffee-substitute, a spoonful of blackstrap molasses in a cup of hot water. One tablespoon of this delicious brew provides your body with not only 3.2 mg of iron but also a wonderful bonus of 131 mg of calcium. Contrast this with the negative effects of coffee. A 1990 study of 101,774 subjects showed that heavy coffee drinking increased the risk of dying of heart disease, even after allowing for other important risk factors such as heavy smoking and high blood pressure.[1] Coffee, because of its acidity, also robs calcium from the bones, contains a central nervous system stimulant that acts as an immune depressant afterwards, and is suspected of being a possible carcinogen. It has been discovered that heavy coffee drinkers have higher levels of cholesterol than those who drink more moderate amounts.[2] Soft drinks also contribute to bone loss when they contain phosphoric acid.[3]

One cannot escape the flood of advertisements extolling the virtues of calcium. Yes, of course, calcium is important, but why is it that the strongest bones are found in the people of the world who supposedly have the "worst" diets? And why is it that the people who eat the most dairy products have the highest incidence of osteoporosis?[4] And how did it get ordained that cattle were to be the suppliers of our calcium? Why not horses, or dogs, or whales? If it's protein you want, rat's milk has much more protein than cow's milk. When you stop to think about the purpose of a species' milk-producing glands, it seems obvious that it is to supply its own newborn with a uniquely formulated sustenance until it can get food on its own. Each species has a different amount of protein, depending on how fast the infants grow. Human beings are unique in that we are the only species that drinks the breast secretions of another species.

Although the returns are not all in yet, it appears that our Western high-protein diet is a major culprit in draining calcium out of our bones. A high-protein diet is highly acidic, and the acid must be neutralized by the calcium stored in our bones. This coupled with a sedentary lifestyle predisposes us to a condition of weakened, fragile bones, just as muscles atrophy from lack of use. It is frequently said that someone fell and broke their hip, when in fact their hip broke and then they fell. Or it is said that someone just sneezed and broke a rib. There's something drastically wrong here, since it seems logical to assume that our bones are supposed to last a lifetime.

There are studies that show that vegetarian women have stronger bones than meat-eating women.[5] Tennis players have much denser bones (by thirty-five percent) in their tennis-playing arms versus their non-playing arms. Both tennis players and swimmers had greater bone density than their non-exercising control counterparts.[6] These studies alone are convincing evidence that both diet and exercise are important in growing and maintaining strong, dense bones.

It is frequently said that genetics plays a role in the incidence of osteoporosis. This is true to the extent that we are predisposed to the effects of too much protein in our diets or too little exercise. There are other studies, however, that show that when people from Africa (with strong, dense bones) migrate to the U.S. and consume the typical Western-type diet, they start showing the effects of osteoporosis.

There's also the myth that pregnant and lactating women need to drink milk in order to grow strong, healthy babies and be able to provide them with enough breast milk after their birth. Since a majority of the world's population has never consumed dairy products, it seems ridiculous that the medical profession as a whole still so actively promotes the consumption of dairy products. In addition, there is a great deal of evidence that cow's milk causes many problems—such as a high incidence of allergies, diabetes, middle ear infections, food sensitivities, constipation, and too much protein in the child's diet, leading to precocious sexual development.

So, what's the role of something like an Ironman Triathlon in osteoporosis? Can you think of a better way to build strong bones than to exercise in three sports? Swimming and biking, in spite of being low (or no) impact sports, still require that muscles pull on bones. These forces are enough to keep bones strong and counteract the effects that tend to tear bone down.

There is a principle that students of anatomy and physiology learn called "Wolff's Law." This says, in effect, that bones grow as strong as the body needs them to be. This means that bones are active, alive, and constantly remodeling themselves, and are, in fact, among the most active tissues in the body. Osteoclasts are cells that tear down old bone, and osteoblasts are cells that build new bone. These processes cause a continuous exchange of bony material in response to the demands that we place on them.

Even more effective in building bone mass, however, is running, although its effects seem to be limited primarily to lower body and spine. Since the most serious fractures from osteoporosis are in the hips and spine, running should be the most efficient exercise to counter the effects of osteoporosis, or preferably to build strong bones and prevent the disease from ever occurring.

As an aside here: Running also promotes healthy disks, the little gelatinous cushions between each of the vertebra in the spine. You've probably heard frequently about "slipped" or "ruptured" disks. For years it was thought that this was what caused so many back problems. In actuality, it was usually weakness of the muscles whose job it is to support the spine. Running helps strengthen these muscles. Diet also plays a role here as well. When the tiny capillaries get clogged from eating an animal-based diet, the blood supply is cut off and this causes ischemia (pain). This is the same mechanism that causes chest pain during a heart attack.

It was recently discovered that running also causes a "loading" of the body's weight on the disks as the body impacts the ground. As it springs off the ground for the next stride, there is an "un-loading." The effect of these loading forces is the "pumping" in of nutrients and oxygen and the removal of metabolic wastes and carbon dioxide. As a result, most runners have strong disks and back muscles. There are definite hormonal influences on bone modeling and remodeling as well as the positive effects of Vitamin D. Since most of us can do little about our hormone status and don't care to get more sun exposure than is necessary or convenient, diet and exercise are the two most viable options to develop and keep strong bones.

Another interesting aspect of how marvelously these human bodies are put together has to do with the intestinal tract taking what it needs from the food as it passes through. For example, it is known that when the body is anemic, more iron is absorbed from the food passing through the intestinal tract. This is measured by a test called the TIBC (the Total Iron-Binding Capacity). When we need more iron, we absorb more. There is, however, no neat little test like the TIBC to tell us how much calcium we are absorbing, but we know that when we need more calcium, the body absorbs more. This explains why women in Africa who get only 200–400 mg of calcium a day have strong, dense bones after twenty years of multiple pregnancies and long lactation periods.

Calcium Pill Deficiency?

For all the reasons noted above, we know that osteoporosis is not a calcium pill deficiency and that we don't need calcium pills to build strong bones. Additionally, studies have shown that giving calcium pills to people who already have osteoporosis does no good. According to a 1996 study by Kanis, even adults who gorged on high-calcium foods did not lose less bone than those with a low calcium intake.[7] Post-menopausal women are frequently given estrogen to try to slow down bone loss but not all women can or want to take estrogen. I'm a good case in point. Because my type of cancer is estrogen-receptor positive, this means that taking estrogen would be like adding gasoline to the cancerous fires. Natural progesterone can reverse osteoporosis without the risk of breast or uterine cancer and is even thought to be helpful for breast cancer patients.

As a precaution I do have annual bone density measurements and, apparently, my regime is working. I'm at the top of the charts as far as bone density for women my age with readings that exceed that of the average thirty-year-old woman at peak bone density. The reason I call osteoporosis the "hidden handicap," is that so many women from the age of thirty-five on are going around with bones that are losing a significant amount of density. They have no idea they are heading for fractures, height shrinkage, rib cages resting on hipbones, and dowager's humps.

In my case, during a period of three years I had a number of stress fractures—

nine to be exact. Skeptics could say that my system was not working, and I have to admit that I questioned my regime at first. After a little research, however, the consensus seemed to be that I was over-training. In my eagerness to improve, coupled with my love of running, I was racing the week after doing as stressful an event as the Ironman. One year I set a new State record in a twenty-five kilometer race the week after doing an Ironman. I was racing every weekend.

No wonder I was having stress fractures, many medics said. I was not getting nearly enough recovery time. In fact, a general rule of thumb is to take one easy training day for every mile of strenuous racing. I've never been able to come even close to that. After the fractures, my energy levels continued to be high and everything else recovered quickly. Ever since, I've backed off on hard runs soon after hard races. I've had no more stress fractures.

Another interesting fact about fractures is that once one is healed, a "callus" is formed at the site of the break. It keeps that site stronger than the surrounding bone for years. I never had to worry about recurring stress fractures, only about how many bones weren't able to take the load I was putting on them. It's now been many years since my last stress fracture and my bone density tests show very dense bones, increasing significantly from age fifty to sixty. The actual bone density of the average thirty-year-old female at peak bone density is 411 mg/cm^2, and mine went from 447 mg/cm^2 age fifty to 466 mg/cm^2 age sixty!

In order to insure that I do get adequate calcium and all the other minerals that go into making bone, however, I do eat mineral-rich foods daily. In addition to the blackstrap molasses trick, I also eat a lot of green leafy vegetables, even adding them, as I said, to my oatmeal in the morning! In fact, if a day goes by that I haven't had a large serving of broccoli, I'll have it the last thing at night.

High Protein Can Mean Weak Bones!

One of the other dietary factors in osteoporosis relates to America's long-standing love affair with protein. For years now, foods have been marketed as being "High Protein" because the label helped sell them. There are high protein pills, high protein powders, high protein cosmetics, high protein anything and everything!

So, what happens when you eat too much protein? What happens is that you go into negative calcium balance as the body tries to compensate for the excess amino acids. The body draws calcium (which is a base needed to offset the increased acid) out of the blood. To replenish the supply in the blood, the body in turn draws it out of the bones.

Occasional excess is not critical, but when people eat high protein meals twenty-one times a week, the effect is cumulative. For example, the Eskimos have a high intake of protein and up to 2,500 mg of calcium a day, and also have an extremely high incidence of osteoporosis at a very early age. Women in their twenties have been diagnosed with osteoporosis.[8] A single fast-food burger, with its high protein, high sodium, and low calcium content, can cause the loss of 22 mg of calcium.[9] Numerous studies support these findings and also the reverse—that plant protein does not cause calcium excretion.

Men, too, are not immune from the effects of osteoporosis. Although it usually starts later in life for men, osteoporosis can still be a very crippling disease. It can cause falls, leaving a person with a fractured pelvis and totally bedridden. Once a person is bedridden, they have no weight bearing on their bones which, in turn, rapidly accelerates bone loss. This can cause a downward spiral impossible to reverse.

These losses are not insignificant. Astronauts returning from a trip in outer space have measurable bone loss. Knowing this, they make an effort to get enough exercise in space to counteract the effect on bones. Shannon Lucid, for example, exercised an average of 2.7 hours a day while in space.

Take heed and know that your bones are another good reason to get a lot of exercise and eat right!

Chapter Seven

Arthritis:
Diet Does Make a Difference

One of my central presumptions is that this body of mine is fairly average and that it responds to good and bad things done to it just as your body would. While I recognize that there are individual differences, there is, as I suggested earlier, much more that is similar than different among us humans. We could not otherwise all have the same blood tests done and show "normal" ranges, and radiologists would be surprised each time they looked at x-rays. And we know this is not usually the case. We are all very predictable.

We all are aware that arthritis is a fairly common malady. We hear pronouncements from the Arthritis Foundation; we read articles in newspapers and magazines about arthritis; and most of us know people who are afflicted with this painful joint disease. What we are told is that it's a rather common affliction; that it's an expected part of growing old (at least in the degenerative osteoarthritic form); that there's no cure; and that diet does not affect arthritis one way or the other.

When I hit forty-two years of age, I went to see a doctor because of the gradual onset of a stiff, painful back. Waking up in the morning, I could hardly bend over. I had to use both hands hanging on to the wall to lower myself down to the toilet, and it took about ten minutes of gradual movement to loosen my back enough to put my shoes on.

X-rays were taken and a hands-on examination was performed. The doctors' verdict was that I had osteoarthritis. I was told it was nothing serious and just a part of growing older. My running, the doctors said, was probably aggravating it and I should just resign myself to the inevitable. They added that there was nothing I could do to help it, but did say there was a new medication, a non-steroidal anti-inflammatory called naproxen, which should ease the discomfort. It was not a cure I was told, and would only treat the symptoms. I was probably going to have to take it the rest of my life.

The pills were great! I woke up each morning able to move without pain, totally flexible, and thought wonderful things about the miracles of modern medicine. During the ensuing years, I'd periodically be asked by doctors if I was on any medication, and I'd usually say that I wasn't because I didn't even think of naproxen as a medicine. Taking naproxen became such a "normal" part of my life that it was just like taking vitamin pills. Then came the medical emergency (described in Chapter Seventeen). The doctors at the Emergency Room at Tripler Hospital asked me the standard question and I gave the standard answer: no medications.

It was only after that diagnosis of anemia that I called my "diet" doctor, John McDougall, to tell him where I was and that the doctors were blaming my vegan diet for not providing enough iron. After all, they "knew" that red meat gave you "heme iron," the "best" source of iron. Dr. McDougall reassured me, saying that if I was suffering from iron-deficiency anemia, I could be sure I was losing blood somewhere. His guess was that I was having gastrointestinal (GI) bleeding. I told him I did bleed periodically from hard or long races. He then said, "You aren't taking any medication, are you?" I started my automatic reply, when I suddenly realized my error.

"Whoa, yes!" I said. "I completely forgot about naproxen. I've been taking that for years now."

"Why in the world are you taking that drug?" he asked.

"For my arthritis!" I replied.

"You don't have arthritis," he said. "It went away when you changed your diet. It's probably the naproxen that's causing your bleeding!"

I immediately stopped the pills, anticipating the return of the painful, stiff back of pre-naproxen days. To my surprise and delight, there was not even a hint of pain or stiffness. When I discussed this with Dr. McDougall, he was not the least surprised. He stated, "Despite what the Arthritis Foundation claims, diet does make a difference!"

Apparently, when I made the dietary changes due to the cancer, inadvertently I did the best thing possible for my arthritis. A recent study has shown that the common non-steroidal, anti-inflammatory drugs, like the one prescribed for me, work by inhibiting the hormones called prostaglandins. This process can actually cause the opposite effect! It can destroy more joint tissue than the arthritis itself.[1] Another interesting fact is that the incidence of arthritis follows the same pattern described earlier with regard to all the common diet-related cancers. Inflammatory arthritis is most common in those countries that eat a high-fat diet and is rare in those countries on a low-fat diet. And, again, it's not because of heredity, because when those people migrate to the U.S. and adopt our high-fat diet, they soon get arthritis at the same frequency as the people around them. What's more, it's even been shown to be true with rheumatoid arthritis.[2]

The theory as to why this happens has to do with the reaction of the animal proteins in our bodies. As these foreign proteins enter our bloodstream, our body's immune system forms antibodies against them, as they would with any foreign protein. In people prone to arthritis, these "immune complexes" are filtered out of the bloodstream and end up in the joints. Here they act like tiny slivers of wood, causing the pain, swelling, and inflammation of the joints. In the ensuing years I have had no arthritic symptoms in my back or anywhere else—and this after a medical prediction that I would be on arthritis medication for the rest of my life.

I also believe that the strenuous exercise program I'm on helps. When the muscles supporting both sides of a joint are weak, they create too much stress on the joint surfaces. Conversely, when muscles are very strong, they support the joint structures and protect them from unnatural wear and tear. In his book, *Aerobics*, Kenneth Cooper talks about the importance of having strong abdominal and back muscles to support the spinal column.[3] Running will do that and was responsible for the elimination of the terrible backaches I had in the years before I started a running program. Of course, there are other exercises that strengthen the back and other joints. All you need to do is find one you enjoy, eliminate all animal products from your diet, and you may cure all your joint aches and pains!

Chapter Eight

Body Fat or What
the Scales Don't Tell You

Most people are obsessed with their body weight. You hear it in their discussions about food, dieting, weight loss, calories, exercising to burn off fat, etc. You can see it in the television commercials, newspaper and magazine articles and ads, and in the supermarkets. Much of our food industry centers on food that does not do what it is supposed to do—that is, nourish our bodies. Unfortunately, being overweight is linked to a host of debilitating health problems, including heart disease, cancer, stroke, diabetes, and hypertension—most of the major killers of American (and Western) people. People in this country spend $33 billion a year trying to lose weight.[1] Nearly seventy-five percent of us is overweight to some degree, and approximately fifty percent of us are on a diet at one time or another. Every study shows that we are getting fatter and fatter.

At the supermarket you see "low-cal," "lite," "no-fat," and lots of photographs of skinny models or line drawings of impossibly thin bodies. Most people seem to be able to eat more than they burn off. Those excess calories get converted to body fat, much to the dismay of youngsters, oldsters, men, women—everybody!

Even a lot of people who don't even look overweight are, in reality, "overfat." This is because the body tucks all those excess calories into muscles as well as the more obvious fat deposits along the waist, hips, abdomen, and thighs. When you look at the profile of a person with a large belly you are looking at a lot of fat! It's first packed around the internal organs, putting pressure on the abdominal wall until it bulges out. The excess fat is also packed between the abdominal wall and skin, making the wearer very uncomfortable as well as unattractive.

We have already talked about which foods to eat to provide maximum nourishment to the body and fill the stomach but not lead to obesity. But when it comes to losing weight, it's important to understand the concept of body fat percentage, not body weight. All body weight that is not fat is considered lean body mass—that is, primarily, bone, muscle, and water. So, if someone is fifteen percent body fat, they are also eighty-five percent lean body mass. (15 + 85 = 100)

This becomes important when diet and exercise are considered. As I said earlier, a low-calorie diet burns off muscle as well as fat, especially if no exercise accompanies the weight loss. It will also drastically lower the basal metabolic rate, the number of calories used in maintaining minimal body functions. This means you will put fat on faster if you resume your previous eating habits.

On the other hand, exercise can help retain the lean body mass while burning off body fat. It will also help keep the basal metabolic rate up. This is especially important to you in the long run, because you don't want your body learning how to become more efficient in hoarding calories. Take two people, both of whom weigh 150 pounds. One may have a body fat percentage of five percent and the other fifty percent. In this example, they will look radically different. The five-percent person will look very lean with good muscle definition, veins obvious through the skin, and contours that suggest a body with very little subcutaneous (under the skin) fat. The fifty-percent person, on the other hand, will not look at all lean. The muscles will be hidden under layers of fat, no veins obvious through the plump skin, and contours that suggest roundness, obesity, and lack of muscle tone.

These are two extremes. What about people who range from twenty to forty percent fat? What do they look like? Well, it may surprise you, but a person with twenty percent fat may look just like the person with forty percent. A lot depends on the distribution of that fat. If much of the fat is in the muscles, then that person could look quite lean. You cannot tell by appearance alone.

Well, What Should I Weigh?

What about all those weight tables and charts that tell you what you're supposed to weigh? Well, you already know enough about body fat percentages to see that they and your bathroom scales don't really tell you what you want to know. Don't throw them out yet, though. They are both useful in giving you guidelines and a benchmark to start with.

Since it is unlikely you will have convenient access to your body fat measurements, your scales can be the first to tell you are gaining weight. Now,

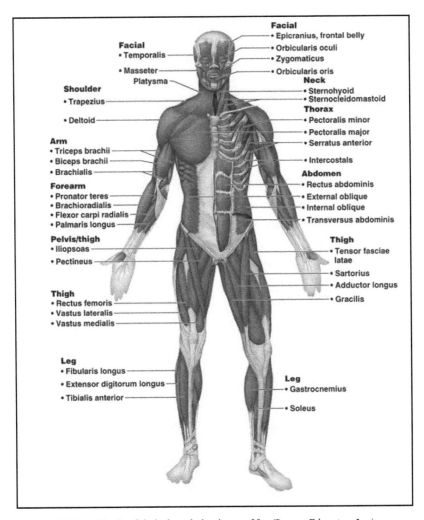

FIG. 3. *Muscles of the body with the absence of fat. (Pearson Education, Inc.)*

since muscles weigh more than fat, how do you know which you are gaining? Unfortunately, if you are eating the typical Western diet and leading a sedentary life, we can both bet that the weight gain represents fat. Your clothes will also be providing clues as they get more and more snug!

If, however, you are not taking in excess calories and are exercising at least three times a week for a minimum of twenty minutes (the minimum required to switch your body to a fat-burning mode), you can still show an increase on the scales. This time, however, your clothes will provide the clue. They will fit better, draping over a much sexier torso. If you want to see what your body looks like with no excess fat, look at the anatomical chart of the muscles on the previous page. You have all those curves inherently; all you have to do is get rid of the fat that conceals them.

So, how do we know how fat we are? There are more than a dozen scientific methods of measuring body composition. Most of them, however, are limited to clinical and research laboratories, or the meat industry. Unfortunately, the most accurate are the most unavailable and most expensive.

Potassium[40]

Measuring the isotope, potassium[40] (K^{40}) is the most accurate method to date, although there are a number of techniques that are being researched now that have been used to measure body fat. Unfortunately, the K^{40} method requires a lead-shielded room and a lot of very expensive equipment to measure minute amounts of gamma radiation.

Electrical Impedance Measurement

Another body fat measuring device estimates the amount of lean body mass by measuring electrical conductivity. This method is convenient, fast, and not horribly expensive (around $20 to $50) but, unfortunately, it is not very accurate. Although it's supposed to be accurate to within plus or minus six percent, it seems to do a better job of measuring hydration levels in the body (how thirsty you are). The subject is supposed to fast for twelve hours prior to the test, consuming no alcohol or caffeine. Also, during the previous twelve hours, there should have been no exercise, subjects should not have gone to the bathroom within an hour of the test, and women should not be menstruating. The subject should also lie still for fifteen minutes before a reading is taken. The electrical impedance varies, depending on whether it's going through lean body mass or fat, and an estimate is based on the measurement of a tiny electrical current passing through the electrodes placed on hands and feet. It's been popular at some running events and triathlons as weight-loss-oriented businesses try to entice new customers.

Near-Infrared Interactance

One of the newer methods is near-infrared interactance (NIR). A tiny light beam enters the body through a light wand placed on the biceps. The presence of fat changes the spectrum of the light beam. The read-out is quick (about ten seconds), cheap ($5 to $25), but not yet widely available. The accuracy range is supposed to be plus or minus three percent and is not affected by previous exercise or hydration levels. There is a major assumption made in the test, however, that cannot be supported. By taking one measurement (the biceps), it is assumed that the fat percentage at that site correlates highly with total body fat in all people. This is highly unlikely as anyone who has done much body fat testing will tell you.

Calipers

The most convenient and inexpensive, but unfortunately the least accurate method of assessing body fat, is the calipers. These look like large pincers, which is, in fact, exactly what they do—pinch the fat under the skin. This method requires an expensive, well-calibrated set to be accurate; not the cheap, plastic kind usually seen at health fairs. You also need a well-trained person to do the testing. The test consists of gathering a fold of skin at anywhere from three to nine sites on the body, measuring their thickness with the calipers, looking up the sum of the measurements of the folds in a chart, and coming up with an estimate of total body fat percentage. The primary areas of inaccuracy stem from the fact that this method measures subcutaneous (under the skin) fat and not any of the fat "marbling" our muscles. (You've heard of "marbled steak" as being the most tender. Now you know why!) It also cannot measure any of the fat packed in the abdominal cavity around our internal organs, producing what we in Hawaii call an "opu nui" or large tummy.

Moreover, people are genetically programmed to store fat in different areas, much to the dismay of women with their "riding breeches" method of storing fat. The margin of error for "skin-fold" testing is supposed to be plus or minus 3.5 to 5 percent. The major value of skin-fold testing, however, can be in its use as a baseline. Once initial measurements are obtained, you can then implement changes in your lifestyle and re-measure periodically to see what results you're getting. The best, and possibly only, solution to excess body fat is to burn up the fat stores through exercise and a slight but definite deficit in calories.

Liposuction

There is another solution—liposuction—that will work, but which many people feel is rather drastic. Besides being very expensive and a surgical procedure with its attendant risks, liposuction is highly dependent on the skill of the surgeon doing the procedure. It requires the judicious application of large and small cannulas (suction tubes) which suck tunnels through the fat. The operation is risky in that you can end up with ridges appearing on the body's surface.

There are other risks as well, such as asymmetry when bilateral (both sides of the body) procedures are done. You could end up with flabby, loose skin. There have also been a number of deaths reported in association with this procedure. Again, you are much better off using a low-fat, plant-based diet and a vigorous exercise program.

Hydrostatic Weighing

The last method of body fat measurement to be discussed is the so-called "gold standard" of estimation, hydrostatic weighing. This entails weighing the person under water. The theory behind this method is based on Archimedes' Principle which states that an object immersed in water loses an amount of weight equivalent to the weight of the fluid which is displaced. By submerging an individual on a sling that is attached to an autopsy scale, we can get a weight measurement that determines body density. Through a sophisticated mathematical formula (using regression equations) and the fact that fat has a density of 0.90 gm/cc and non-fat body tissue (lean body mass) a density of 1.10 gm/cc, we come up with a fairly reliable method of determining body fat percentages.

The disadvantages to this method are that it's not readily available, it's fairly expensive, and the person has to be able to expel nearly all of the air from his or her lungs while underwater. A lot of people have trouble coping with that. Additionally, a source error exists in the lungs and the gastrointestinal tract. A very expensive gas dilution system is needed to determine accurately the residual lung volume, and a high-fiber, gas-producing meal can give you an inaccurately high reading!

Getting it Right

An accurate estimate of body-fat percentage can be of crucial importance to an athlete. Rapid weight loss by an already lean, muscular individual can cause severe degradation in athletic performance. More importantly, when muscle is broken down, high levels of urea, ammonia, and purines are released into the blood and can cause kidney damage. When muscle is lost in an adult, it is also much more difficult to replace. In a sedentary individual, it will never be replaced and leads to a higher proportion of fat. This, in turn, leads to less calorie-burning tissue, causing the person to gain weight even easier than before.

As I have said, this is why I never recommend fasting or very low calorie diets. We want just enough of a calorie deficit to cause the body to burn fat, not muscle. It will burn muscle when it is in a starvation mode, or even just "thinks" it is starving. And it will "think" it's starving when it doesn't get enough calories!

This is one of the most critical points to remember whenever you are tempted to try a calorie-restricted diet, no matter how highly acclaimed it is.

So, how much fat should we carry around? You've probably heard that we must have some fat to survive. It serves several purposes such as insulation, padding, and energy storage. When you consider, however, that the average thirty-year-old woman is thirty percent fat, you can guess that there's more than enough here. The average thirty-year-old man is nineteen percent fat, so again, there's lots to spare. Compare these figures with the average long-distance male runner at from four to nine percent fat, or the female distance runner at from six to twelve percent fat. Ironman triathletes tend to possess a little more body fat than other runners, probably due to the fact that swimmers in general carry more body fat. My own experience is that training bouts lasting eight to ten hours create an enormous appetite, and I have to eat a lot to sustain the energy levels required to complete that many hours of heavy training. I notice that I can really "pig out" and still lose weight. The eating part is the most fun part, too!

Chapter Nine

Starting an Exercise Program

O*kay, okay,* you say. "I'm convinced! I've known for a long time now that I need an exercise program but I just haven't known how to get started." Or maybe you're one of those who is an ex-exerciser. You know what to do; you just haven't been doing it. Or perhaps you're a sporadic exerciser. You are gung-ho for a while and then get away from it. Then, when you're ready to start back, you have to go through all the aches and pains of just getting started again.

No matter what condition you're in, the first thing you need to do is plan. In order to plan, however, you need to know your present level of conditioning. If you're a rank beginner, we have to start you at a very low-level program. And the ideal program is cross-training—two or three sports that will work out all parts of the body and not overstress any one set of muscles.

Get Checked Out First!

Assuming you're average or normal (and they are not the same thing) and have not exercised in a while, you should get a physician's clearance. This is to rule out any hidden problems that could surface as a rude surprise. This is especially true if you're over thirty-five or forty years of age. A physical check-up would also be a good idea if you're young and have never really exercised—the type who escaped physical education classes for any one of a number of possible reasons, or if you have always been exercise-phobic. Once you've been declared basically healthy and cleared to start training, you need to assemble a number of pieces of equipment.

Getting a Running Start!

The easiest sport to start with is running. You'll need a pair of running shorts, a running singlet or T-shirt, and a pair of running shoes. While it is possible to start with sneakers and regular sports clothes, it is important to be comfortable and avoid possible injuries. Non-running clothes can chafe and bind; and sneakers will probably not give your feet the support they need for running. Go to a running store and try on several types of running shoes. Many will let you do a short run so you can check out the fit of the shoes. The mistake most people make is to buy shoes too small, so make sure there's plenty of toe room.

As you get more into the sport, you can add niceties such as visors, sweat bands, fancy time-pieces to calculate splits and running pace, and tights to keep your legs warm in cooler weather. You can also have warm-up suits for before and after running, a headset radio to keep you company in areas where it's safe to run with one, water bottles to keep you well hydrated, and elastic shoelaces to save you time and effort in putting on and taking off your running shoes. You may also get heart-rate monitors that range from ear clips to finger sensors, to straps around the chest that send telemetry data to a sensor at another location. There are new gadgets out on the market all the time and some of these are very useful. You'll want to evaluate these on your own. You may find that some of them add to the challenge and enjoyment of your workouts.

You Don't Need a New Set of Wheels

For the beginning cyclist, things get a bit more complicated. You're fortunate if you already have a bike. You don't need a fancy racing machine to start off with. In fact, it's better to wait until you know what you want. For the time being, almost any bike will do. You will probably need some professional help on fitting the bike to you. Adjustments, higher or lower, can be made with the seat and stem heights. I'm afraid no bike is going to be comfortable for the beginning cyclist trying to go for long rides. You will probably hurt in places you never suspected you'd ever hurt!

A few simple modifications will turn any old bike into a pseudo-racing machine. Add one or two water bottle cages to prevent dehydration—a real danger on long rides. You can unscrew the conventional pedals and add toe clips or clipless pedals that will add immeasurably to your riding safety, speed, and comfort. A racing saddle won't do much for comfort for a while, but it will be better than the old spring models that a lot of cruiser bikes are equipped with. If the bike has upright handlebars, change over to the racer's drop handlebars.

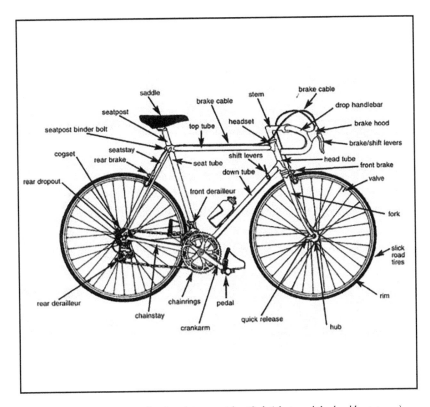

FIG. 4. *Your "racing machine" with its parts identified. (platinumbikeplan.blogspot.com)*

If you want to go all the way, change the gear clusters so that you can do steep hills, add racing wheels to lower your rolling resistance, and add triathlon-style handlebars with elbow pads that put you lower on the bike for a more aerodynamic position. All these modifications can wait, however, until you've had a chance to see how much you enjoy cycling, how competitive you want to be, and how much money you want to put into the sport.

In addition to the basic set of wheels, you will need a safety-approved helmet. It is crucial that you start out with one since you're most apt to fall early on as you're learning your bike-handling skills. As a matter of fact, falling is a risk that even the cycling experts face because, even if you were perfect, not everybody else is! So, play it safe and protect your most valuable asset, your brain.

The rest of the cycling equipment is primarily for comfort. For the body, get padded cycling shorts, a cycling jersey, cycling gloves, and cycling shoes. For the uninitiated, a properly outfitted cyclist makes quite a sight. The shorts are skintight, have chamois (or simulated chamois) padding in the crotch, and come mid-way down the thigh to protect the inner leg from chafing. Luckily, though, cycling shorts seem to be the "in" thing to wear now.

The cycling jersey is also skintight and has funny little pockets around the back. After an hour or so on the bike, you'll learn how convenient these pockets are for food, sun block, and more food. As I've said, the bike should be equipped with water bottle cages; but for really long rides, you'll want to stick an extra water bottle in one of the pockets.

Cycling gloves are funny looking, fingerless, padded, and colorful. They are fingerless to allow the unencumbered use of your fingers and padded to help absorb road shock through the handlebars and for when you and the road meet unexpectedly. Cyclists' shoes come in two versions: touring and racing. Touring shoes look almost like regular shoes except that the soles are more rigid, and there are ridges across the center of the soles to hook into the raised portion of the pedals. You can then get off the bike and walk like a normal person. Racing shoes make you walk funny, just the opposite from tip-toes, due to the cleat which locks into the pedal. These are a little tricky getting used to, but once you've made the conversion you'll never go back. Implicit in this is another good reason for always wearing a helmet. Novice cyclists (and even some old hands) sometimes can't get out of the cleats in time and find themselves unceremoniously dumped. Embarrassing but survivable!

The next accessory you'll want is for the bike. There are little bags, usually with Velcro straps, that attach to the bike under the seat (called the "saddle" by serious cyclists). In this little kit you'll want to be prepared for flat tires. Add a set of Allen wrenches, a little crescent wrench, a spare tire or tube, a patch kit, some pre-moistened towelettes, and money for a phone call in case all else fails! (You can read more about bicycling in Chapter Eleven.)

Getting Your Feet Wet

Swimming requires only a bathing suit, goggles, and water. Most serious female swimmers wear one-piece suits and swim caps, both for aerodynamics (or is it hydrodynamics?). Men wear the non-boxer swimsuit and swim caps for the same reason. Hair, seams, and floppy material slow you down.

Goggles are necessary whether you train in the ocean or a pool to protect the eyes from salt and chlorine, enabling you to see continuously in the water and out. In fact, some of my most enjoyable ocean swims have been off Waikiki Beach where you can see where the underwater lava flows from years ago ran into the ocean. You also need to see well above the water line so that you can navigate accurately. So, get good goggles. There's nothing more miserable than hard plastic jabbing you around the eyes, unless it's goggles that fog up. My longest swim thus far has been five miles, and while I hurt in a lot of other places my head wasn't one of them.

There are other miscellaneous training aids that can help allay the boredom of swimming pool laps. These include: hand paddles, pull buoys (foam cylinders which go between your legs up at the crotch to raise the lower body and enable you to concentrate on your arm stroke), kick boards (to allow you to concentrate on your kick without having to worry about your arm stroke), and a number of resistance gimmicks, such as a swim suit with pockets like a parachute and elastic bands tethered to the end of the pool so that you can swim forever and never have to turn around. (Read more on swimming in the next chapter.)

Keeping Track

The last two items needed before you start are a waterproof watch that can measure seconds, and a journal, fancy or simple. There are any number of exercise log books on the market. Check the "Running" section of any bookstore. Keep track of your type of exercise, heart rate, comments about the day's exercise, and then weekly totals. An optional item that adds considerably to the fun of checking your body's "tachometer" is a heart rate monitor. This will make getting readings faster and more accurate and can conceivably keep you from getting into trouble, which you'll know if your heart rate gets too high.

The journal will be useful now and in the future. I find mine useful as I thumb back through years past to see how far I've come. The journal should be able to record a year's worth of data, such as the time and distance for each of the sports, the heart rates associated with each, and a column for comments.

Checking Your Pulse

Now that you've got the basic equipment, we need to do an assessment of where you're at. Start with taking your resting heart rate by counting the pulse at your wrist or neck for one minute. Now, nobody I know has the patience to stand there for a whole minute, so just count the beats for ten seconds and multiply that figure by six, or you can count six seconds and add a zero. To get the greatest accuracy, start your count with "zero."

Record this figure in your journal. If you're average, your resting heart rate will be around seventy-two beats per minute (bpm). Generally speaking, this heart rate will give you an indication as to how aerobically fit you are. The lower the number below seventy-two, the greater the fitness. And, of course, if your heart rate is higher than the average, just think how much improvement you're going to see!

Next, calculate your maximum heart rate. There are a number of ways to do this but the simplest is to subtract your age from 220, the theoretical maximum that you were born with. Let's assume that you are thirty years old; your maximum would theoretically be 190. Now, let's calculate your training intensity range. Take sixty percent and eighty percent of 190 (multiply by .6 and .8). This gives you a range of from 114 to 152 bpm. This tells us that anything under 114 bpm is probably not intense enough to give you a beneficial cardiovascular training effect and that anything higher than 152 bpm may be too intense and that you're courting injury. This training range gives us workouts in any of these three sports that will yield aerobic (with oxygen) benefits and subsequent improvement in your cardiovascular condition.

The heart rate then gives us the information we need to determine how intensely we should train. The next question is how long. We need to get a baseline measurement that will be determined by how fit you are at this moment. And your fitness level will vary with each sport. You will need to find a course to measure swimming, biking, and running distances accurately. An example in my local area is the twenty-five-meter pool where I do some of my swim training, a fifteen-mile route around that area, and a 400-meter track at the university.

To get your baseline measurements, swim four lengths of a twenty-five-meter pool (100 meters) and note the beginning and ending time. Later, when fully recovered, bike a fifteen-mile loop (or some such distance) and note that time. Again, when fully recovered and preferably on another day, run a mile (four times around a 400-meter track), and note that time. Now you've got some baseline measurements. Also, get your heart rate measurements at the end of each of the three trials. These should not be done on an "all out" basis. Do each of these at a comfortable, but not too slow pace.

It's a little difficult to get your heart rate while doing each of the three sports without a heart rate monitor, but you can stop and immediately get the count to give you an idea of the range your heart is operating. You will soon get a pretty good feel for where your heart rate is relative to your level of effort. If you're rolling along very comfortably, hardly breathing hard, you can be pretty sure that you're at the lower end of sixty percent, whereas if you're "dying" and panting hard with eyes darting wildly, you are more likely operating at or over the upper end of the training range. You will soon learn when to push yourself a little harder and when you need to back off on the pace.

Some people have difficulty in finding their heart rate, especially if they are swimming or on a bike. According to one of my physician friends, there is a good correlation between heart rate and breathing rate. What this means is that you can count breaths per minute rather than heartbeats per minute. Find your normal breathing rate. This is your baseline and/or fully recovered rate. Then check your breathing rate at the "rolling along comfortably" rate described in the preceding paragraph. This will be within your aerobic envelope, the range at which you want to do most of your training. Don't bother with checking out your maximum, please. That will be past the aerobic threshold and into pain! We don't want you exercising there until you are superfit and going for age-group records.

Planning Your Exercise

You may find that these "trial" distances are where you need to start, and that one or more may be too short or too long. For example, you may not even be breathing hard by doing the 100-meter swim. In that case, do 200 or 300 meters. Stop at the point where you feel you are just starting to feel fatigue, measure your heart rate (or breathing rate), and record it. As for the bike test, you may just barely be able to get through fifteen miles, in which case you can drop the course to ten or even five miles.

The same applies for running. It may well be that one mile is a good distance for you to start. If so, you can plan gradual increases of from five to ten percent every other week in all three sports. Then look at your personal calendar and decide when and how many days a week you can devote to your training. For example, you may be able to swim at noon three days a week, Monday, Wednesday, and Friday. You may want to get your biking in to and from work, or Tuesday, Thursdays, and a long ride on Saturdays. Running may have to be done early in the morning, after work, or whenever. Just be sure not to go more than three or four days between workouts for each sport. Conversely, don't schedule workouts too close together without adequate recovery time. Elite athletes can train twice a day, but most of us mere mortals cannot!

You now have enough information to plan several weeks of workouts. Example: Week One might consist of swimming 400 meters on Monday, Wednesday, and Friday; cycling fifteen miles on Tuesday and Thursday, and twenty-five on Saturday; and running a mile early in the morning Monday through Friday. At the end of the week, review the week's workouts and make adjustments if necessary.

If you are feeling energetic, strong, and ambitious, you're doing it right. Stay on that schedule for another week (Week Two). By then you should be ready to increase the distances. So, Week Three might look like this: swim 440 meters Monday, Wednesday, and Friday; cycle 16.5 miles Tuesday, Thursday, and 27.5 miles on Saturday; and increase the run to 1.1 miles. These gradual increases will allow lots of time for the body to adapt to the new stresses being put on it and will keep you from getting injured. You'll also be developing a triple-sport lifestyle that will make you feel lean, mean, and fantastic.

By Week Four you'll be able to increase again, assuming that your end-of-week assessments are all still "Go"! Don't be afraid to back off if you are starting to feel soreness or fatigue. But, on the other hand, don't be tempted to jump the schedule by leaps and bounds just because you feel so darned good. That's how many of the "walking wounded" get into trouble!

Speaking of walking, there is a lot of talk about the benefits of walking as a fitness exercise. Naturally, if for any reason you are unable to run, you will have to walk. What you will find, however, is that walking is not nearly as effective or efficient an exercise as running. It is very difficult to get your heart rate up into the training ranges, and it takes much more time to cover the same ground. As long as you have not waited too long to start your fitness program, I recommend starting with slow running. You'll be miles ahead if you do (pun intended)! Plus, you'll burn twice as many calories. Scientific research shows that a 140-pound person burns ninety-six calories per mile running instead of forty-eight calories per mile by walking.[1]

Want a Flat Stomach?

Lastly, consider adding some abdominal exercises and some weights to your weekly routine. Flat stomachs come about when two conditions exist: strong abdominal muscles to support your internal organs and the absence of excess fat deposits. This is where both daily vigorous exercise and the vegan, low-fat diet come in. To strengthen the abdominal muscles, crunches are very effective. Lying flat on your back with your hands cupped lightly behind your head, raise your upper body straight up and hold it for two to three seconds. The exercises that do most for your large muscle groups are: bicep curls, lat pull-downs, tricep curls, squats, lunges, calf raises, and calf curls, both front and rear. Ideally, we all should have access to a well-equipped gym, but you can do most of these exercises at home with minimal equipment. Once your commitment to a lifetime of exercise deepens, however, consider joining a gym or even getting a home gym.

Chapter Ten

Swimming:
How To, Where To, and the Rest

I
f you are like me, you learned how to swim many years ago as a child. You may have been taught by your parents, other kids, or through a physical education class at school, the old-fashioned wheel stroke—that is, arms slicing straight down through the water.

Because I learned to swim at such an early age, breathing coordination was never a problem. It's only when I'm coaching new swimmers that the subject of breathing efficiently comes up. There are several basic principles beginning swimmers need to keep in mind.

Breathing Efficiently

You inhale between arm strokes in the little trough that forms between your head and shoulder. You pivot your head just far enough to the right or left to get your mouth out of the water, and you inhale on the sideways upturn of the head and exhale on the downturn as your head goes back into the water. Keep your mouth open and exhale through both nose and mouth. This keeps water out of the nasal and oral passages. Well, most of the time, anyway. Once in a while a wave breaks at just the wrong time and you'll gulp a mouthful. Just figure that you're getting a free sip of fluids and keep on going!

Can you imagine the shock I felt when, as I started to train to do triathlons, somebody told me I needed to "learn how to swim"? Here I'd been on the swim team in high school and had even been a swim instructor and lifeguard, and now I was having to learn this new stroke. It was not quite as bad as learning how to walk all over again, but almost.

Fortunately, colleges, YMCAs, and recreation centers frequently offer swim classes. I signed up for one and saw a film demonstrating the "proper" arm stroke, which entailed bending the elbow at a ninety-degree angle and moving the arm in a slight "s" stroke. The theory goes that you need to keep "new" water moving. The old straight-through stroke just moves the same water and does not move you ahead as fast as when you are sculling from side to side and grabbing new water continuously, much like a propeller moves through the air. On the second day of the course, we were videotaped and shown what we were doing. Then we were taught the new method and videotaped again. What a difference! Although it felt very awkward at first, it was not long before there was no question in my mind that this was a much better way to swim. The other shock I had was to see how low in the water my legs dragged. Once I saw that, it was no trouble to change my kick and tilt my pelvis so as to keep my legs and feet close to the surface. My swim times began to drop immediately. So, if you are of the old- or no-school of swimming, get yourself to a good swim coach and learn the most efficient stroke. It'll pay dividends right away.

If you're a more recent vintage swimmer, you're already ahead of the game and will just need to get back into a good training program. In this sport, as in most others, the social aspects can be very important. I always found that training in a group with a good coach was fun!

Even Adults Need Toys

In the last chapter I covered the basic equipment required for swim training. I recommended getting the "toys" that go along with swim training such as pull buoys, kick boards, fins, hand paddles, etc. They can help relieve the boredom of swimming laps in a pool, which is where most people have to train.

The ocean is nice to swim in, but most people do not have access to it, and it is almost impossible to measure and time your laps. In this sport, as in most others, the importance of feedback cannot be underestimated. Positive reinforcement gives you joy and pride in your progress, and if you can't measure your progress, you're at sea, literally and figuratively.

There is one disadvantage I've found to doing all your training in a pool. Your back muscles get a rest every twenty-five or fifty meters (or yards) as you scrunch up to push off against the wall of the pool. Then when you have to do a long swim in a triathlon, your back muscles are unaccustomed to having to hold that same position for the half-mile, mile, or 2.4 miles required in a standard Ironman. Another skill that you need to train yourself in is to navigate while swimming. You cannot just rely on the black line at the bottom of the pool, because not too many triathlons with open-ocean swims have underwater course markers. I've actually seen it one time; a mile swim course at the Wailea Triathlon on Maui had a line on the ocean floor that traversed the entire swim course.

Barring that, though, it's amazing how many people add a lot of distance to their swim by heading off in a different direction from where they intend to go. While you can just lift your head to see where you're going, it ruins your form and speed. You can't always depend on others for your navigation, either. I've seen whole packs of swimmers go off course during a race. You may notice, while swimming, that if you have to cough, you'll have a tendency to do it underwater rather than while your face is out of the water, grabbing a breath of air. Your lungs always have some residual air in them. You cannot exhale all the air from them, even if it feels like it. If, however, you cough underwater, you are tapping into that residual air, which throws off your breathing rhythm and makes you feel as if you need to gasp for air. You may have to break the nice, smooth pattern of your breathing to get more air sooner. This is better than going into oxygen debt. Try to keep as much oxygen going to the muscles as possible by keeping the lungs as full as possible.

If you're doing a triathlon, it's very important to orient yourself at the beginning of the swim leg in ocean swimming. Being off just a few degrees can add minutes and fatigue to the swim leg in a race. Pick a tree, a building, anything that you can see while you're in the water to aim for. Once in a while during a rough ocean swim, the waves can be high enough to make it difficult to see your landmark. That's when you check ahead to see where the other swimmers are, keeping in mind that they may be having trouble, too. In this case, go with the majority until you have evidence to the contrary.

Another tip to keep in mind is when you're doing ocean swim legs in events that have course turns marked by buoys. Sight the buoys as soon as you can, aim directly for them, and cut the corners so close that you actually brush the buoy. Of course, you may find that a lot of other competitors are doing the same thing. Charge on ahead and get through the choke point as quickly as possible.

A skill that will also help you in navigation, balance your upper body muscular development, and distribute your fatigue is that of bilateral breathing (breathing on alternating sides). Most people learn to breathe on one side or the other and feel that the non-favored side is very awkward. Once swimmers consciously change the pattern of their breathing to alternating sides, however, it soon becomes second nature. As you alternate your breathing sides, you will always know where you are and can make continuous course corrections.

Of course, you do need to keep your eyes open. I would not normally think this an obvious thing to mention until one day I was talking to my favorite training partner, Kate. After Kate's first Ironman distance ocean swim off Waikiki, I remarked on the beauty of the lava flows through the sand off Diamond Head and all the beautiful fish we'd passed. She revealed for the first time her fear of the ocean. She'd had to swim almost the entire 2.4 miles with her eyes squeezed shut!

Kate is by no means unique. There are a fair number of brave souls who have to conquer agoraphobia (fear of wide-open spaces), fear of sharks, plus normal healthy fear of the hazards of open water swimming. Boats and other over-water craft have trouble seeing swimmers in the ocean. In addition, they are not used to having to look for them.

Swimming Safely

For this reason, always wear a brightly colored swim cap and keep a constant watch for all types of watercraft. Always swim with a buddy, although there unfortunately is nothing that precludes both of you from getting run over, as has happened. Safety is another good reason to develop the skill of bilateral breathing as it enables you to keep an eye on everything around you. Just don't forget to keep casting your eyes about and even behind you as boats and other watercraft can quickly overtake you.

Avoiding Boredom

One aspect of pool training we all have to deal with is the boredom associated with just going back and forth. As I'm preparing for a training session in a pool, this thought comes up frequently. There have been a couple of times when I've gone to the pool and been unable to swim, for example, after several of the surgeries I've had when the doctors have not allowed me to swim before the stitches were taken out. Sitting there watching the people go back and forth, I'd think how boring that must be.

Then, one day, after an enforced lay-off, I got back into the pool and I started concentrating on the many aspects of my stroke, responding to the frequent exhortations from Ricky, my swim coach, to get my elbows higher. All of a sudden I realized that an hour and a half had passed in a flash. I then understood that what the out-of-the-water observer sees bears no resemblance to what is actually going on under the water!

A Word about Wetsuits

Swimmers have discovered that the higher in the water they can swim, the less the frontal resistance. The less the frontal resistance, the faster they go. Well, wetsuits are buoyant and, therefore, keep you higher in the water. So, you will see lots of swimmers in warm, tropical waters as well as the chilly waters of northern climes wearing wetsuits. A wetsuit will also prevent hypothermia, the lowering of your body temperature, too. So, at times, it is a piece of safety equipment. It is a definite asset to the swimmer's closet.

Even if you never intend to become a triathlete, swimming is one of the best forms of exercise. It is excellent training for your cardiovascular system, it stretches you out; and it's gentle on your body. It's a sport you can do for the rest of your life, long after you might have to give up cycling and running. So learn to enjoy it, and do it as close to daily as possible. If you have a lot of weight to lose, it may be one of the only aerobic exercises you can do until you get your weight down.

Chapter Eleven

Bicycling:
Getting Mechanical

One of the things that makes the cycling leg of a triathlon unique is that it is the only leg in which failure can be attributed to a piece of equipment. After all, you can run barefoot if you lose your shoes; you can swim without goggles if a strap breaks or you lose them; but you cannot do the cycling leg without a functioning bicycle.

For the mechanically challenged, getting on an equal footing with your bicycle can be pretty intimidating. I've seen young, macho men look at a derailleur (gear shifter) and recoil in horror. On the other hand, I've seen "fashion-plate" women with long, red fingernails dig right in with wrenches and come out with the greasiest, dirtiest hands you ever saw. The point is: Anybody can learn the basics of bicycle mechanics.

The most fun way to learn how your bike operates is to sign up for a course on cycling. In many parts of the country, you can find a course called "Effective Cycling."[1] It's rigorous, well organized, and sanctioned by a national organization that insures the course is well taught by licensing their instructors.

Besides learning about bike operation, you also find out what to look for in buying a bike, how to fit it to your body, how to ride in traffic, simple and complex repairs and maintenance, safety maneuvers, bike touring, and much more. Another benefit is that you get to meet the nicest people!

Upon completion of this or a similar course, you will have been transformed into a confident, competent cyclist. You will know your rights on the road and how to merge safely with automobile traffic. You learn things like watching a car's front wheel to know which way and when it's going to turn. You learn "bail-out" maneuvers, panic stops, and even how to fall properly when all else fails.

Caution: Be Careful!

Now, if I've made cycling sound a little dangerous, know that it is. There's no question that there's a great deal of risk involved in placing yourself on the roads where the automobile has been king for so long. Many motorists tend to view cyclists as invisible, petty annoyances who belong on the sidewalk or playground and who have no right to impede their automobile's progress down the road at breakneck speed.

There are even aggressive motorists who, when screaming insults and narrow misses don't seem adequate, will literally try to run you off the road. National and local cycling organizations are grappling with these problems through educational and legislative efforts. Both approaches are slow and have many obstacles in their way. For example, the time to teach cycling is when kids get their first bikes. They are now taught haphazardly and sometimes erroneously—for example, when they ride against traffic. But trying to get cycling into the school curriculum, which many consider already overfull, is difficult. Most people don't realize that through cycling kids can learn physical fitness, the basic laws of physics, courtesy, nutrition, and independence, and gain a mode of transportation that frees them from the tyranny of automobiles for the rest of their lives. Idealistic? Perhaps. When you consider society's dependence on fossil fuels, the pollution of the air we breathe, and the fact that our kids are growing up obese and very unfit physically, you can see how the lowly bicycle can transform society in some very positive ways.

In Hawaii, traffic congestion has reached near-panic dimensions. People have to get up earlier and earlier to get to their jobs on time. People joke about paving the island over with freeways and parking lots, except that it's not a joke anymore! Lifestyles in "Paradise" have been modified to the point where most people would be hard-pressed to see any difference between living in Honolulu and Los Angeles—except that Los Angeles has more bikepaths! If more people would get on their bikes to ride to and from work and school, they could relieve the congestion on the roads and reduce the need for parking lots. They would also save lots of money, get the exercise/training in during the time they'd ordinarily be sitting in a traffic jam, and arrive at work or school feeling wonderfully invigorated instead of fuming and irritable.

Don't Sweat the Sweat!

A little sweaty, you say? Just where do I shower, you want to know? That's not a problem! If you start out with clean clothes and eat a non-animal-food diet, your sweat doesn't smell bad. It's the breakdown of animal products that causes the typical meat-eating society's characteristic body odor. And besides, you're using a different set of sweat glands when you're exercising.

We humans have two different kinds of perspiration glands. One set of glands, the eccrine, secretes moisture to cool our bodies and carry off some of the waste products of our metabolism. The fresh sweat of exertion has very little odor. It is only after bacterial decay sets in hours later that you get the typical "locker room" smell, and this is generally from clothes that have not been laundered soon enough. The second set of sweat glands is the apocrine, the set that does not generally operate when we exercise. It's the apocrines that start functioning when you reach adolescence and give off that musky, mate-calling scent we try so hard to mask with deodorants.

So, after your commute to work or school, you can always go to the washroom and take a sponge bath. A quick change of clothes, a comb through your hair, a little make-up if you're a woman (although you certainly won't need to add that nice, healthy glow to your complexion since you'll already have it!), and you bounce into the office feeling wonderful! If you're a little fearful about appearing "odd," try to talk some of your work pals into riding with you. Then cycling is absolutely fun, and the bonding that occurs between people while riding gives you a head start on all your relationships at work. There are all kinds of benefits to be realized.

Beating Gridlock Traffic

Depending on how far from work you live, you may get all your training in at no extra cost in time. If you get really enthusiastic about riding, you'll be out on the roads on Saturdays and Sundays, too. If that's the case, you'll have no trouble getting in lots of training miles. If you're like most of us, however, it's a little more difficult getting those miles up to where we want them. Even if you ride to and from work, it still might not be far enough to get the total weekly mileage you need for triathlon training. That's when long weekend rides are a must. Try to find a bike club with a group of riders who are at or a little above your competitive level. Not only will you get some good training, you will improve rapidly and you will have the safety of riding in a group.

We've discussed training goals in a previous chapter whereby you establish how many miles a week you need to ride, but you also need to look at different types of rides. You can break the rides down into two basic types, endurance and interval training. Endurance consists of training your legs, heart, and lungs, and, as we say in Hawaii, "okole" (rear end) to hang in there for the long haul. As a beginner, that may be twenty-five miles, but for the old-timer that could also be 200 miles!

Don't make the mistake I made in my early days of training. I thought that cycling was just a matter of getting on the bike and pedaling, and that I could go on that way forever. I certainly found out differently when, at the end of my first triathlon bike leg, my rubbery legs could hardly support my body, much less run. A weekly long-distance ride will probably handle the endurance part of your training. To take care of intervals, you need to set up a training program consisting of getting out on a road with little or no traffic once or twice a week, along a pre-measured course, and doing a workout consisting of periods of hard cycling, followed by recovery. Your heart rate will tell you how long and how hard you can go.

Checking the Heart Rate

Start out by going very hard for a period of time measured by a watch or cycle speedometer. As your heart rate approaches ninety percent of maximum, back off until your heart rate drops down to sixty or seventy percent. Then repeat the process three or four times. I guarantee you will have an excellent workout.

If you don't have a heart rate monitor, it'll be more difficult trying to measure your heart rate the old-fashioned way. But you'll soon get the hang of it, as your pounding heart will let you know it is being pushed. When you can no longer feel that pounding and your breathing starts to approach normal, you can guess that it's time to go again. If this doesn't sound like a lot of fun, it's probably because it isn't. This is the part of my training program that I have the most trouble with. This is another case where working with a group helps provide motivation.

We've already covered a little in Chapter Nine about modifying your old "clunker" into a racing machine and why cyclists wear what they wear. Cycling technology is such that there is always new equipment out on the market. It doesn't take long to get on the mailing lists of the mail order catalogs of bike houses so you can see the latest equipment. It's also a good idea to subscribe to at least one cycling magazine to provide periodic updates and receive a monthly dose of motivation.

Because cycling relies on a piece of mechanical equipment which has a tendency to fail on occasion (usually the worst possible moment), view each of your (and your cycling mates') mechanical failures as an opportunity to learn and rehearse what you'd do in a race. If your buddy is an old hand at fixing flats and you're still terrified at the mere thought of it happening to you, you'll ingratiate yourself forever when you offer to change his or her flat. Don't even mention that, in return for this favor, you expect some tutelage; that usually is never in short supply. Then as you finish getting that rear wheel through the maze of the chain, cog, and derailleur, you'll be unbelievably proud of yourself. What's more, you'll have lost that fear of having a flat under extreme pressure. You'll know you can handle it.

There are lots of other things that can go wrong. As you pile up the bike mileage, you'll be exposed to them first or second hand. Never miss an opportunity to stick your nose into the middle of a mechanical crisis. Even if you've studied the problem and handled it in the past, you can probably still benefit from the review and help teach others at the same time. You'll feel so much more comfortable on the bike if you know you can handle the common malfunctions that will catch up with you sooner or later.

Chapter Twelve

Running:
Getting Fast and Staying Uninjured

R unning can be as simple as putting one foot in front of the other and leaning forward. It can also be so extremely complicated that it takes a computer to analyze all that is going on in the body as it moves from point A to point B in a ballistic fashion.

I started running back in the days when there was not a great deal published about running. In fact, it was at a bookstand in July 1968 that I saw a strangely titled book called *Aerobics*[1] by Kenneth Cooper, M.D.. I'd never seen the word before (Dr. Cooper had just coined it), so I picked up the book, thumbed through it, and noticed that it referred to the effect of different types of exercise on the body. I bought it, and got so engrossed that I read it in one sitting. In the book, I found the definition of aerobic exercise and how it affected every body part and system, literally from head to toe. At the grand old age of thirty-three, I was plagued with a horrible assortment of maladies such as two ruptured disks, insomnia, constipation, and high blood pressure. With each chapter that I read, I found a possible solution to a health problem and was anxious to try exercise.

The easiest of all the exercises described in the book was running. It was also the most effective and efficient. It took no special equipment, and it could be done alone, any time and any place. It seemed ideal for me. The next morning I went out for my first run (in tennis shoes!) and have been hooked ever since. Learning nearly everything the hard way means that it seems as though I've experienced almost every injury a body can have. Since then, I've read almost everything dealing with running I can get my hands on. I've always found the subject fascinating, and it seems research keeps supporting the need for lifelong exercise.

How much do you know about running? If the answer is "Not much!" then all you need to know, for now, is to put one foot in front of the other, lean forward, and don't do too much. How much is too much? Your body will let you know. For beginning runners there are all sorts of signals from the body. Foot pains, chest tightness, "shin splints," sore quadriceps (thigh muscles), etc., will be the messages from the body that something new is going on. At that point, you just back off a little. You don't have to stop; just slow down. You may even need to walk for a while, but do keep moving. Keep track of the time and/or distance covered and be consistent in your program. For starters, schedule an hour a day, preferably first thing in the morning. This way you get it over with, your energy levels will be charged up, and emergencies, minor crises, and temptation(!), will not call a halt to your program.

Now, you will not necessarily be running for the full hour. You will run according to your fitness level and walk to round out the hour. A great rule to remember is: Run until it hurts; walk until it doesn't! If you can run for only ten minutes the first time out, that's okay. Walk for the rest of the time. The next day start again at ten minutes or whatever level you ran at the first day. If body parts are hurting, stop at ten minutes. If nothing is complaining, go for fifteen minutes. Or if you go around the block the first time, go two blocks the next time. If you're just starting an exercise program, set your goal for twenty-one days. Let nothing interfere with this scheduled time, which will preferably be first thing in the morning. The reason for the twenty-one days is that it takes that long to establish a habit pattern firmly. The reason for the time—first thing in the morning—is that it gets the job done! There is no interference and no procrastination. Studies show that the most successful exercisers are morning exercisers.[2]

The main points that must be remembered are: Be consistent and increase slowly. If you do both right, the body will complain a little bit but not too much. If you're an old hand at running, both principles still apply. I believe everybody needs daily exercise, so belong to the daily school of running, modified in the following way. One day hard or long; next day easy or short. That's why keeping a log is so important. You need to monitor your intensity and distance so that you don't overdo it and still keep improving.

Make It Hurt Just a Little But Not Too Much!

If you keep your body totally comfortable, it could be because you're not increasing the stress on it. And if you're not increasing the stress on your body, you're not getting stronger. So, a little discomfort is a good sign. Remember: Run until it hurts; walk until it doesn't! You also need to insure that you don't overdo it and get yourself injured. The rule of not increasing your distance by more than ten percent a week or month is pretty safe, when you get to reasonable levels such as a mile or two a day.

So, how do you know how much is "too much?" Other than pain signals, your log or journal will offer an excellent way to keep track of your training. I sometimes feel that my training is much like juggling three or four balls; I barely get one ball into the air and another is about to fall. I finish one sport workout and another is almost overdue. The only way I know where I stand in each sport is by keeping a running tally in my log.

Another measure I find valuable is my weekly total workout hours. By monitoring this I can pick up trends in my training hours' totals (unfortunately, usually downward). By keeping weekly totals relatively constant, I know that the demands on my body are within range.

The equipment needed was touched upon in the chapter on starting an exercise program. The main points to remember are that you need good shoes (good quality with not too many miles on them, but not necessarily anything fancy), comfortable clothing (nothing that chafes or binds), and a source of water. Running can cause you to sweat a great deal, and it only takes a very small percentage of fluid loss to cause real dehydration problems. This can cause not only loss of performance but also disorientation, possible permanent kidney damage, and lots of things you don't even want to consider having happen to you.

That's why you need water. How much? Remember this tip: It takes about eight swallows to get enough fluid in the stomach to activate the pylorus, the valve that opens to let stomach contents into the small intestine. This is where the water starts getting absorbed into the blood stream. Here's another test: your urine should be clear. If it's not, you need to drink more water. Remember the C3 rule: Clear, Colorless, Copious!

If you're an average adult, you probably have a fairly decent running form. Most people's feet track fairly straight along the line in which they're moving. Their arms hang loosely from their shoulders with elbows bent at about a ninety-degree angle, and move easily back and forth in rhythm with their legs. And most people are fairly relaxed in their lower arms, neck, and head. If, however, you're not average, you may have some type of running-form abnormality. It's always a good idea to find a running coach and have your running stride analyzed.

A good coach can quickly tell you if, for example, your head is cocked to one side, or you are carrying your arms too high, or you are throwing your legs out to the side as you run. The real pros have their forms analyzed by computer, although if you have an abnormality it may well be that you are compensating for some variation in your body's center of gravity, which is changing constantly as you run. If this is the case, there will be no need to change your running form. Just be sure to have someone look at you from time to time to be sure that no odd little quirks creep in that could cause you injury or slow you down unnecessarily.

Running Is Not Boring!

The most frequently asked questions a runner gets asked is, "Don't you find running boring?" And the answer is, "Not even close." Besides thinking about the training I'm doing, my mind tends to cover a myriad of things, and I sometimes find that an hour may have passed with my hardly being aware of it. Put me with a group of people, and I am laughing, joking, solving my/ their problems, and feeling wonderfully close to them as a result. Sometimes, although not as often, we just run together in silence, just sharing the feelings of our bodies hard at work.

As your running mileage increases, you will find that your mind either associates or dissociates. This means simply that you stay mentally tuned into your running or you go off somewhere else. I find that both happen to me. I start a run associating. I think about a slow, gentle warm-up as I gradually increase the heart rate and get cold, tight muscles to gradually loosen and warm to the task. Then I slowly increase the pace but never to a point where I'm uncomfortable.

After a while my mind starts to wander. If I'm bothered by a problem, it'll start gnawing at me and, very often, a solution presents itself. This is also a wonderfully creative time for me. Ideas keep popping up in my head, sometimes so many that I really get excited. Usually, however, by the time I get home, most of them have evaporated. I've taken to running with the micro-cassette recorder that my daughter, Laurelle, gave me for Christmas so that I can capture these ideas. In fact, many of the ideas found in this book were created "on the run," so to speak. I found that if I didn't capture them at that moment, there were so many that I couldn't remember them all. I've found that there's nothing so fragile as an idea, and nothing so fleeting. This feeling of being mentally stimulated, of being able to solve problems, and having wonderfully creative thoughts has a basis in fact. When we are exercising aerobically, the brain is getting extra oxygen. Not only is there a short-term stimulating effect on thought processes, but there is a long-term effect in the form of increased blood circulation. The brain develops larger, cleaner arteries and more capillary formation. As a result, aerobically fit people think more clearly and creatively.

Running Is Not Bad for Your Knees

The second most frequently asked question has to do with running being bad for your knees. This is a myth that prevails because people think that cartilage wears out. Animal protein can sometimes trigger an autoimmune response that can cause the body to attack its own cartilage.[3,4] Running actually helps build cartilage, as I mentioned when talking about arthritis (see Chapter Seven). The compression during the weight-bearing stage squeezes out the blood from the tiny capillaries; then when you're airborne, the blood rushes back in, pushed by the increased blood pressure from the running.[5,6] Nearly 500 runners were observed over an eight-year period and found to have developed only a fifth as many knee and leg problems as non-runners. Women reaped the most benefits with almost ninety percent fewer knee problems than their non-running counterparts.[7]

Another thing to keep in mind is the "talk test." You should run at a speed that is slow enough that you have enough breath to carry on a conversation. If you're huffing and puffing while trying to talk, you're on the edge of anaerobic (not enough oxygen) running and need to slow down.

Running training in general should be aerobic (with oxygen). It's only when you have an adequate mileage base—say, thirty to forty miles per week—that you can begin to think about anaerobic training. These would be your intervals at the track, for example. When you get to this stage in your running training, join a running group. In Hawaii, we have several excellent coaches who conduct running sessions at the local high school or university tracks. And I'll bet that almost any area has some good coaches, if you just look around.

Once you join a group, you'll find that your running will improve dramatically. You will find, first of all, that your enjoyment of running increases, which alone tends to encourage your running. More importantly is the discipline that regular sessions encourage. The structure imposed by a coach and a regularly scheduled meeting time is invaluable.

Coaches are also important information sources. As you increase your running distance and intensity, you may be faced with various aches and pains. It's important to know which ones signal a need to back off in order to prevent injury. It's also interesting to note that we can tell ourselves something, but it never seems to have as much credibility as someone else telling us that same thing. So, get a coach!

Running as an exercise or sport seems to just "grab" some people, while for others it's a crushing bore. For those like me who love it, the need to increase one's longest run distance seems to be almost insatiable. When you do your first ten-kilometer run, you think about fifteen kilometers. Then you start to think about marathons and ultra-marathons. Marathons and longer distances, for some, have an appeal that is exciting and challenging. As a runner crosses the finish line of their first marathon, they usually think one of two thoughts. They may think, "There, I've done one and I'll never do it again!" Or, they may think, "Wow, if only I'd trained a little better, I could have knocked off ten or (fill in the blank) minutes off my time!" After a period of recovery, they may start thinking of running marathons in different locales. As I have discovered to my joy, marathons are run literally all over the world.

Programming the Mind

One of the comments that I hear most from people is that they cannot imagine running a marathon as the third event of the Ironman. As a matter of fact, when I had done my first 100-mile bike ride, the way I was hurting I could not even conceive of *beginning* a marathon. The major difference between that first 100-mile bike ride and my first Ironman is mental programming. In other words, when I climbed on the bike that first morning, I "knew" that all I had to do was that 100 miles. That was why I didn't collapse at fifty miles, or eighty miles, or any distance less than 100 miles. On the other hand, that morning of my first Ironman I programmed my mind to do a 2.4-mile swim, a 112-mile bike ride, and then a 26.2-mile run. Now, you have to have done the physical conditioning to enable the body to support the mind in accomplishing that goal. I knew, for example, that in spite of feeling intense fatigue at the eighty-mile mark of the bike ride, I still had a marathon to go. I did not give my mind any choice in the matter.

The goal was set. The body had been sufficiently trained to support that goal; and the rest, as they say, was history. As a matter of fact, I have never *not* finished a race. I may have given up on setting any records for a given race, but I've found that I can always dig a little deeper. To me, finishing a race has always been more important than anything else, and the positive reinforcement gained from finishing just keeps that behavior going. I recall that at the twenty-two-mile mark of my first marathon, I "decided" I would never again put myself in that position of such extreme discomfort. About that time a nice, good-looking young man came up along side and started running with me. He, too, was "dying." Just then, I got an idea. I knew that if we could dissociate for just a bit, we could probably get through that marathon. So I asked him if he wanted to try an experiment to help get us through. He, of course, agreed. I told him to visualize the most exciting erotic experience he'd ever had, or would like to have.

He looked a little surprised, smiled, and said, "I got one!" He shared his, and I shared mine, and the next thing I knew, the finish line was in sight and we sprinted for it. That taught me a bunch! At about that same point in the marathon of my first Ironman, I recalled that experience. I was feeling totally depleted and wondering how I was ever going to finish. I then dropped back to the person behind me who turned out to be a friend.

Duke was absolutely miserable. His running shoes had been lost at the transition from his bike, and he'd been offered someone else's shoes in a desperate, last-ditch effort to save the race. Duke had not only trained hard for a year for this event, he'd also traveled all the way from Saudi Arabia, where he was stationed in the Army, just to compete in the Ironman. The shoes were way too small, and Duke was bloodied and almost beaten. We started dissociating and, of course, you know the rest. There never was a more welcome sight than the Ironman finish line that day!

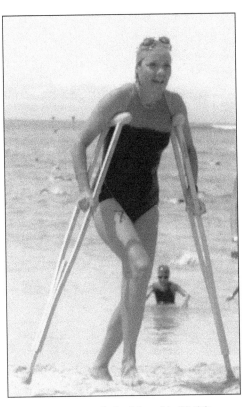

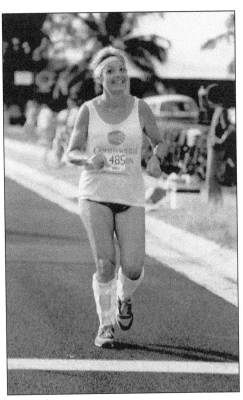

Coming up on the finish line of the Waikiki Roughwater Swim two weeks after pelvic fracture, September 3, 1984. **PictureMan**

Completing a half-marathon three days after diagnosis of two (bilateral) tibial stress fractures, May 8, 1987. **PictureMan**

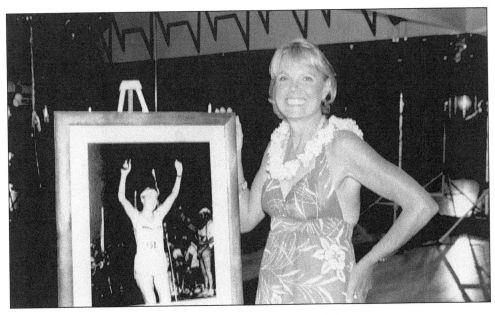

Being inducted into the Gold's gym's "Hall of Fame," October 1997

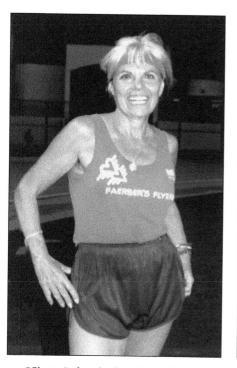

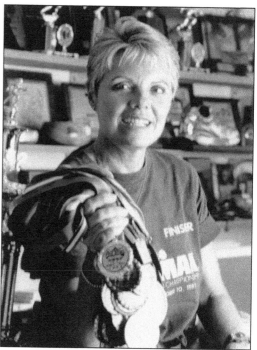

"Glowing" after a hard workout at the track,
January 1998

With some of my medals

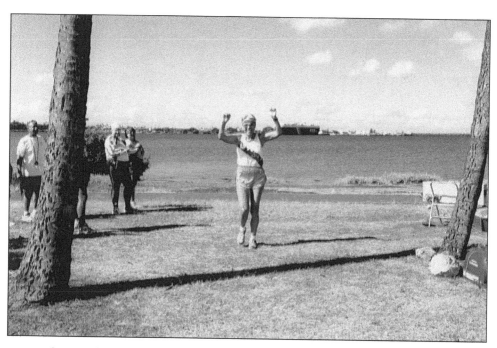

Coming in first place at the Pearl Harbor 10K, with Pearl Harbor in the background. August 2003

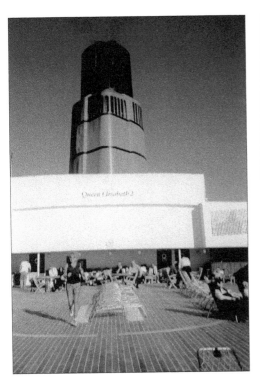
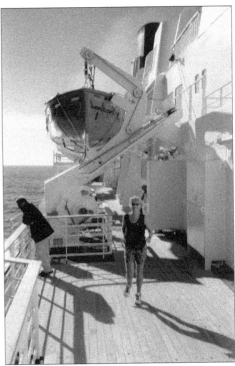

Running on board the Queen Elizabeth II, mid-Atlantic. September 2001

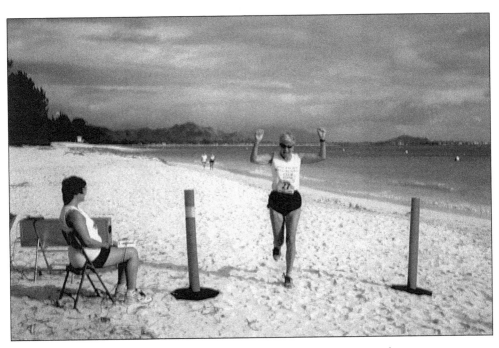

Finishing first place at the Kailua Beach five mile race, Kailua, Hawaii. July 2003

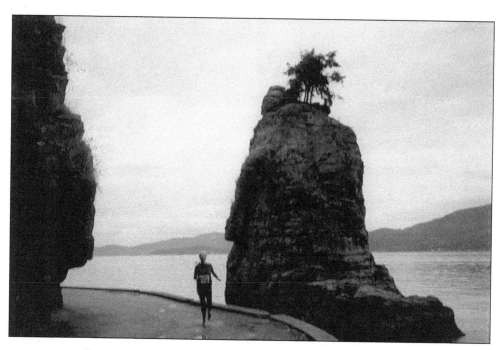

Running at Stanley Park by Siwash Rock, Vancouver, B.C., Canada. February 2003

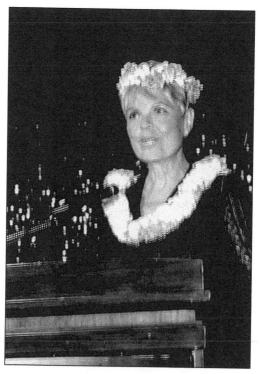

Giving the keynote speech for the opening of the Breast Care Center, Holy Cross Hospital, South San Francisco, CA. November 2005

Chapter Thirteen

Putting It All Together: You're Running a Marathon

S o now that you've got three sports handled, are you ready to do a triathlon? Well, you could! These athletic events are so much fun that you'll rarely see the competitors without smiles on their faces. Well, most of the age-groupers, anyway. Age-groupers are usually the middle-of-the-packers who are there because they enjoy the sport and want to do well primarily when stacked up against their age-group peers.

Let's face it. If you're over forty, you really don't have much of a chance against a well-trained twenty-five-year-old. So to keep the action lively for everybody, you get to compete in age groups, usually with a five-year spread, e.g., 20–24, 25–29, 60–64, 90–94, etc. You will always find male and female divisions as well. If you get an age-group first place, you'll know you did very well when stacked up against athletes who are much more closely your equals.

Advantages of Cross-Training

Aside from the fun of the competition, I believe that multi-sport training is better for the body. Each sport tends to emphasize only certain muscle groups. These muscle groups can be overworked, leading to injuries, and leave other muscle groups under-exercised. Because training is extremely muscle-specific—that is, no other muscles get exercised and trained—multi-sport events cover more of the body. Running emphasizes the hamstring (back) muscles of the legs; cycling, the quadriceps (those bulging front thigh muscles); and swimming, the shoulders, chest, and upper arms. This is not to say that no other muscle groups get exercised, because they do. It's just that they don't get exercised with nearly the same intensity.

When you put all three sports together, you get an excellent overall body workout. All three sports contribute to cardiovascular fitness and all three are excellent fat-burners. I've seen both men's and women's bodies totally reshaped into pleasing, curvaceous contours. And you can bet that the owners of those reshaped bodies are darned proud of their new forms. Those clinging aerodynamic outfits have more than one function!

So how does the human body cope with all these different demands placed on it? Very well, thank you. Sure, there are muscle groups that tighten up while doing one sport, but they get loosened and stretched in another. Blood vessels open up in response to the increased demands made to support the greater blood supply to the muscle groups being used. This happens automatically; and just as automatically, the blood switches to the second, third, or whatever are the next sets of muscle groups being used.

This is why I have found that it doesn't matter in which order you do your training. Blood vessels are two-way streets, so to speak, and they will shift to wherever the demand is. I have done back-to-back workouts in every conceivable order and have found that the transition is easy. As a matter of fact, although the swim is usually first in a triathlon, I love to finish my training with a swim because I'm cooled down and stretched out. It's the best way to end!

The Importance of Transitions

In a triathlon it is obvious that the first one across the finish line wins. What is not as obvious is that it is not always the fastest swimmer-cyclist-runner who crosses that finish line first. Time is required to switch from one sport to another. This activity is called a transition, which at times can make the difference between winning and not winning. In your workouts you will need to practice transition training. This consists of rehearsing the switching of your swimming gear for cycling gear; and cycling gear for running gear.

The best way to do this is to lay out all your equipment in the transition area, thinking carefully about the order of use. As you're coming out of the water, you'll be pulling off your goggles and cap, and thinking about what you'll be doing when you find your bike—which, of course, you will know by noting the location of a very strategically placed landmark. Races have been lost because of "lost" bikes. Some triathlons start so early that you're placing your bike in a rack in pitch darkness. When you come out of the water, the scene is totally transformed, not only by the setting but also by the sea of bikes. Know your bike location!

Do you want to know how to tell a novice triathlete? They're the ones with the bucket of water to wash the salt or sand off. The old hands know that it's a waste of time to shower or rinse off your feet before putting on cycling shoes. The salt does not cause chafing, and besides you will soon be creating a salt bath with your own perspiration. Don't worry about sand or dirt on your feet from running out of the water barefoot. The sand or dirt will drop right to the bottom of the socks or shoes, and you will never even know it's there. You know that it's much easier to pull on bike shorts before you put on shoes. You'll want to pull on your cycling jersey before you put on your helmet. And you'll want to wait until last to put on your gloves and sunglasses!

All these things suggest the order in which to place your equipment. You'll also want to have a plastic bag in which to put your swim gear. While the protection of the "used" equipment is not a priority item during the race, the scratching of a $30 pair of goggles can cause a lot of consternation long after the race is won.

Upon returning from the cycle portion of the race, you'll need to get out of your bike shoes (unless you're a super-sport who just pulls your feet out of the pedals as you dismount, leaving the shoes still attached to the bike). You can also be pulling off your gloves as you approach the transition area.

Some athletes just run in their bike shorts to save transition time. If it's a particularly hot day or a long run, comfort can be a very important consideration. What have you gained if you've saved fifteen seconds in transition and your pace is five seconds per minute slower because your body is overheating? Since body temperature rises so fast during exercise, overheating is a real problem. A lot of male competitors shed their cycling jerseys for the same reason.

Read All About It!

If you're a serious competitor, you're already subscribing to the sport's journals. This is how you keep up with what's going on in the sport. There have been whole articles just on transitions. These magazines also offer clues to what's new or upcoming in the field of equipment. Your friendly triathlon shop is probably stocked with dozens of little (and not so little) gadgets to help you go faster. It's worth your time doing some serious browsing on a continuing basis and getting on good terms with the store clerks who very frequently are some of the sport's top competitors. As you pick their brains, you'll be picking up valuable tips on all aspects of training and racing. As you find something new and hopefully better, you will need to try it out. It just makes good sense never to do anything different on race day. You will need literally to go through the motions of each transition. When you find the sequence that works best, then you can go through the motions mentally. Visualization is an excellent adjunct to your training. As you're out on long runs, picture in your mind coming out of the water, and how it feels as your legs re-adapt to weight bearing on a vertical plane instead of horizontal. Your mental checklist should include how you're going to replenish fluids in spite of not feeling thirsty.

All this rehearsal will lead to your keeping a cool head and not panicking, irrespective of the pandemonium going on around you. I use my transition time to calm myself and run through my own mental checklist. You will usually find race volunteers in the area, ready and very willing to assist in whatever way they can. If you need help, ask for what you need in a very calm, specific way. I've seen competitors yelling, cursing, throwing things, with the poor volunteers saying, "'It?' I don't know what 'It' is! Just tell me what you need." Pronouns do you no good if the volunteer doesn't know which "it" you're referring to. In any case volunteers never deserve to be yelled at. They are just as excited as you are and just as anxious to help you get back on the road. Use but don't abuse them!

Now, let's assume you've just gotten through your first triathlon. While everything's still fresh in your mind, write down all the lessons you've learned. If you're smart, you'll never make the same mistake twice. Since most triathletes don't do too many back-to-back races, it'll be some time before you do another one. To prevent those feelings of panic the night before a race, make some notes on what worked and what didn't work. It'll also save you a lot of anxiety as you prepare to do your next triathlon.

Have You Hugged your Race Director Today?

Besides those wonderful volunteers, there are race directors. These self-sacrificing souls also need to be treated right. If things have gone wrong, the race director needs the feedback, but preferably in a calm, rational way. After all, if it's not a satisfying experience for them, they won't be back either. So, negative things need to be broached with constructive comment. What race directors love more than anything else, however, is to know what went well with their race. So be a good competitor and treat everybody well!

Chapter Fourteen

Time Management:
How to Fit It All In

T hrough the auspices of the American Cancer Society's Speaker's Bureau and their breast cancer support group, Reach to Recovery, I've been able to talk to hundreds of people about the value of lifestyle changes in the prevention of and (if prevention is not possible) in the dealing with the diagnosis of cancer.

One of the most frequently asked questions has to do with finding the time to do all the things I've mentioned so far. This issue is one that I faced squarely when I started a running program back in the late 1960s. Since I've always been the type of person who gets involved and who has always worked while going to school, time is extremely important to me. In an effort to squeeze more into every day, I've taken several time management courses and read a number of books on the subject.[1,2] The main principles that I apply have to do with prioritizing things to be done and getting up earlier in the morning.

When I started running in 1968, I was working as a guidance counselor, going to graduate school, and raising and trying to cope with two adolescent kids by myself. As one might guess, any extra time was at a real premium. Yet, after reading Kenneth Cooper's book, Aerobics, I knew then that I had to find the time to add exercise to my life. It also seemed that adding exercise would not only pay off in physical benefits, but would enable me to be more efficient in my work and study.

The only time available to squeeze in my running was early in the morning. By rising an hour earlier, I was able to devote a sufficient amount of time not only to getting a good workout in, but I also found that hour a wonderful time to be alone with my thoughts. I planned my day, solved problems, experienced the joys of watching a sunrise, felt the coolness and quietness of early mornings, and returned from those runs feeling euphoric, strong, lean, healthy, and hungry. After a good breakfast, my energy level was much higher than I'd ever experienced. I knew that I'd found a way to handle all the stress generated from the job, graduate school, and raising kids.

De-Stressing "Stress"

It was in those days that I developed my philosophy of stress. I have found that "stress" is a catchall term too frequently used to explain anything inexplicable. In other words, it's a scapegoat. What I've discovered is that when our bodies are exercised strenuously every day, stress as an entity ceases to exist. Many of the afflictions Westerners suffer are frequently attributed to stress: heart attacks, ulcers, high blood pressure, acne, insomnia, drug addictions, etc., have all been thought, in this country, to be caused by stress. Yet, when people eat a plant-based diet and get a lot of exercise, you rarely find these health problems.

No matter how pressured I was with the demands of a job that required constant "giving" to other people, the pressures of voluminous reading, writing term papers, a thesis, getting good grades—as well as enduring the questionable joys of raising two teenagers—I still had lots of energy. This could only have been done with an exercise program that allowed me to problem-solve and, at the same time, dissipate the tensions and anxieties that kept building up, i.e., stress. I'd always return home from my runs feeling ready to tackle the world. I knew I always had to make the time to get my run in.

I was immediately hooked. I integrated running into my daily routine, making it as much a part of my morning ritual as brushing my teeth. Never was there a thought of "should I?" or "shouldn't I?" I was into running shoes and out the door before I knew it.

To this day, more than thirty years later, I feel the same way about running. The only change has been that I occasionally add a rest day after a hard race. This is only because I've learned that if you don't give the body enough recovery time, it will create it, even if it has to go "on strike" to do it. Rest after a hard effort is just as important as training. It is just as critical for rebuilding new cell structures, whether they're muscle, bone, tendons, or ligaments. I've also become experienced at running through injuries. Adding running to my daily routine has actually bought me time as it has added energy and efficiency to my days. But what about swimming and cycling, you ask? Well, that took a little more planning.

Since I lived about eleven miles from work and have always thought commuting was a horrible waste of time and gas, I started biking to and from work. I have to admit that, at first, it seemed an almost impossible endeavor. There seemed too many problems: What about showering after? What about a change of clothes and shoes? What about make-up and sweaty hair? What about flat tires or other mechanical problems? What about what people would think?

Here I was, one of the few managerial-level women who had enough "image" problems as it was! Did I really need to be doing something that could be considered so unconventional? What about that steep hill I lived on and would have to bike down at break-neck speeds and bike up after a long day's labor when I was tired?

Handling the Gremlins

One by one, I conquered all the gremlins. A sponge bath in the ladies room took care of cleaning up after. I carried a change of clothes and shoes in a backpack. I did my face and hair after arriving at work. I learned a lot about changing flat tires in a hurry and, after a series of flats, I discovered vinyl tire liners, which practically eliminated flat tires completely. Getting home was a different story, since that hill took a lot longer climbing back up, but I reasoned that I was getting some "hill training"—something that builds power in the legs. I tackled the hill in stages. On the way home I had to walk the bike up part of the hill only once, the first time. After a week's biking, it seemed so natural that I wondered how I could have made such a big deal out of bicycle commuting.

I also decided that it was time to give up conducting my life by what people would think. Then I found out that their reaction for the most part was a mixture of incredulity and admiration. Before long, I started seeing more and more people biking to work. This is a trend I would like to see accelerate. As I have said, it's a wonderful way to combine fitness and solve our cities' transportation nightmare. I even discovered that I could get to work in less time than it took me to commute. There was also the time saved in getting workouts scheduled.

Fortunately, the swimming training was easier to solve. There were two swimming pools within a short walking distance from my office. I swam three times a week and in those early days, a half-mile seemed like a lot. As my speed increased, I increased my distance. Then on weekends I did a long (relative to my training level at the time) ocean swim. "Long" used to be a half-mile; now "long" is five miles. It's amazing how our perceptions change.

As I started to get more serious about training and competing, I wanted to add weight training. Looking at my calendar, there were the two other noontime slots, Tuesdays and Thursdays. So, weight training got added to the schedule, and I still had evenings free, except for the weekly track workouts with my coach, Johnny Faerber, and "Faerber's Flyers."

When I had my medical leave of absence after my second cancer surgery, I relished the additional time I felt could be devoted to training. What I found out was that when I had more time, I got less efficient and did not get any more training in. I also found out that the body serves you with a self-limiting alarm. When you try to do too much, it rebels by sending out pain signals. These must be attended to; if they are not, injury is certain to follow.

Setting Goals: Are We Done Yet?

Another way to slice the training "pie" is to train by time. You can go out for one, two, or say four hours, especially if you are in a new locale or while traveling. As long as you know that there is an end, and approximately when that end is, you can hang on. What happens when you don't know when or where the end is, is that you want to give up. In the absence of any feedback, your brain says "This could go on forever!" and then goes into a state of "overwhelm." When overwhelmed, you are too tempted to quit.

In beginning my distance swim training, I selected the half-mile course located at the Ala Moana Beach Park near Honolulu. The waters there are warm and sheltered by coral reefs. The first time, I got in the water at the start and swam for what seemed forever. Progress seemed frustratingly slow as I picked the high-rise building at the mid-point as my point of reference. It even took "forever" once I got abreast of the building itself. When I finally reached the end of the half-mile course, I walked back.

After a couple of months of this, I'd gained enough strength and courage to swim both ways. That, of course, seemed to take the "forever" that the first half-mile did. That was interesting, I thought, as I tried to figure out how to handle the longer distances without giving up.

The Importance of Sub-Goals

Then I discovered that the lifeguard stands were 200 feet apart and that there were five of them. I knew it was no problem for me to swim 200 feet because that was only eight lengths of a twenty-five-foot pool. So I did that and then went for the second 200 feet or lifeguard stand, and so on. Now I swim 2,000 feet so much more easily than I ever thought possible. When I get bored, I just count lifeguard stands and it's never more than just a few until the end. That discovery totally changed my concept of the swim distance.

The same principles apply to indoor bicycle training, which, even in Hawaii, is sometimes a necessity or a convenience. Rather than just get on the bike and go for as long as I can, if I just set some intermediate goals I can get through a workout of any length. Another little trick I've learned is to count by tens to a hundred. By counting to ten on each of my ten fingers, I can get to a hundred repetitions of anything relatively painlessly. This is how I get through doing three hundred sit-ups at a time or climbing up a steep hill on a bike while standing. You can always bear the pain just a little bit longer when the end is in sight.

One-Two, One-Two, Running into Self-Hypnosis

Looking back on my training for the Ironman, I could see that what I was doing was a form of self-hypnosis, although at the time I had no idea of what was going on. First, I'd get into a relaxed rhythm with my running, swimming, or cycling. And, of course, all three of these sports are very rhythmic with their one-two, one-two cadence.

These sports can also be very dissociative. Once you get the mechanics of the running, swimming, or cycling down automatically, your mind will very naturally wander. It was at that point that my mind would start to visualize scenes of triumph and excitement as I could see myself crossing the finish line of the Ironman. What I didn't know then was that I was switching to "right-brain" function.

You may have heard that our brains are divided by neurological functions into right and left sides. The left side of the brain for most people is where we analyze data, have our time consciousness, and do our checking of reality—all the concrete, objective types of thinking. The right brain, on the other hand, is where we create, dream, lose track of time, and are not hampered by any practical limitations. We can transport ourselves anywhere in space and time, from the origins of the planet to far into the future. We can be anybody or anything!

It was in this state that I started to transform the dream of doing the Ironman into a reality. I started increasing the length of my training sessions totally lost in right-brain activity that, of course, also made the training so enjoyable that I'd look forward to the next training session. What I was doing was, in effect, giving myself positive reinforcement. This meant I felt my training was providing me with rewards and other nice things above and beyond anything I was doing for my health.

So the lessons were learned. As your physical training progresses, your body becomes more able to handle the greater distances. As your body is able to handle more, the mind leads the way by setting greater goals, and the lesser ones, by comparison, now seem easy. All you have to do is go along for the ride. And what a ride it is!

People with hectic schedules usually envy those who appear to have more time. They needn't. Busy people are usually more efficient because they have to be organized, prioritize their demands, and develop and follow schedules. I hope that this dispenses with the most common excuse for not exercising. We must find time to exercise, and it will reward us by providing us with more quality time and greater enjoyment of the time we do have.

You're Entitled to 120 Years!

Scientific studies show that our exercise time investment will be rewarded at the end of our life as well.[3] The time spent training is not only added on in terms of living additional years, but it also gives us a greater quality of life to the very end. The ideal is to live out our full life span (said to be 120 years), active, completely self-sufficient, and with all our capabilities.[4] We should be able to die in our sleep with little decline in our physical and mental functions.

More than eighty percent of our population dies of lifestyle-related diseases at ages far below 120. It doesn't have to be this way. You have it within your power to control your life span through diet and exercise, making drastic changes if you need to. Take a look at some of the master athletes in their eighties and nineties and you'll see what I mean. They are spry of step, mentally alert, sexually active, and still enjoying life to its fullest. Can't find any of them? Attend some of the World Vets Championship races and the Senior Olympics and you'll see age groups up to and including the 100s. This exercise and diet program really does work!

Chapter Fifteen

Looking Good, Feeling Sexy

While walking to the start line of a ten-kilometer race one Saturday, I caught sight of Susan, an elite (meaning super-fast) young runner. She, too, was walking to the start line. Alongside her was an obviously in-shape young man. Susan was talking away animatedly and reached out to give him a couple of pats on the behind. I smiled, broke into a little jog, and said as I passed her, "Keep your mind on the race, Susan!" All three of us had a good laugh and an excellent race. (We all won our respective divisions.)

I cite this incident, not only because I smile every time I think about it, but because it illustrates a point. Fitness is sexy. When you feel good about your body, it returns the favor. And when you look around and see a sea of fit, trim bodies, it is sexy. Bodies without excess fat allow firm, curvy muscles to show through. This is true irrespective of the sex and age of the person. We all have the same basic skeleton, the same basic musculature and, therefore, the same potential for beautiful bodies. It's the fat covering up those beautiful muscles that, in excess, makes bodies unattractive.

So it starts with the initial physical attraction. Then, when people run together, they tend to open up and share their thoughts and concerns, many of them very intimate in nature. This creates a strong emotional attachment between two people. This can happen with people you've never seen before and may never see again. But the bond is there. I can remember people I ran with ten years ago, especially if they were encouraging me at a time when I was sagging and needed it. I know it works the other way around, too, because people I have encouraged during a race have thanked me years later.

Along with the initial physical attraction and the bonding that occurs with sharing, is the value system that fit people have in common. Athletes value their bodies, health, and performance, and others who share these values. Conversely, athletes frequently find it difficult to enjoy people who abuse their bodies whether it's by getting fat, using drugs, or just not exercising.

Besides these psychological aspects, there is the physical side as well. A fit body functions better. Fit bodies have stronger hearts, blood that carries more nutrients, iron, and oxygen, and wide-open blood vessels that supply these nutrients to every cell of the body.

Who Needs Viagra, Anyway!

Some male runners have noticed that they have stronger erections as they get in better cardiovascular shape. This is very likely because as the cardiovascular condition improves the blood supply to the penis improves. And since erections are a vascular event, it is likely that, as the vascular condition improves, the quality of the erections improves. After all, erections are dependent on a good blood supply, and a good blood supply occurs as a result of both regular vigorous exercise and a low-fat plant-based diet.

There seems to be a popularly accepted perception that strong erections in men diminish as they age. The hoopla that greeted the introduction of Viagra is evidence that the Western lifestyle is causing erectile problems. (Wouldn't you imagine that a man who had all the erections he wanted would have no need or interest in a drug like Viagra?) The clogging of the blood vessels that supply the penis, and not merely aging, would explain why erectile dysfunction occurs. If the process continues unimpeded, impotence is the result.

The smart man who values the sensual side of life, without the potential negative side effects of taking drugs, has another good reason to eat a low-fat vegan diet and get lots of vigorous exercise.

Keeping a Healthy Prostate

Another positive benefit to men from following this program concerns the prostate. The prostate is a gland that surrounds the neck of the bladder and the urethra in the man. As men in the West age, their prostates tend to enlarge, frequently to the point where their urine stream is greatly diminished. This is something that often leads to a number of urinary tract problems. In fact, most people, including physicians, think an enlarged prostate is an inevitable fact of men's growing older. This frequently means that older men can't empty their bladders completely and, as a result, have to get up during the night to urinate, thus disrupting their good night's sleep.

What's really interesting is that in countries where they eat a low-fat diet, men don't suffer this problem, which, by the way, goes by the medical name of "benign prostatic hypertrophy." Doesn't that sound like a good reason alone to eat a better diet? There's also the fact that cancer of the prostate in men is lower in countries where men eat a low-fat diet.[1]

Women Don't Have Prostates, But...

Since the female reproductive system functions in a similar way (the blood supply to the clitoris, vagina, uterus, etc., is dependent on wide-open arteries and capillaries, too), this is just one more of the many reasons to take good care of our bodies.

Too Tired to Poop?

You may have heard that runners suffer from a diminished sex drive, broken relationships, and all kinds of other problems related to increased exercise. This probably comes from the population of runners who are just beginning and experiencing the pain of the initial phases of an exercise program. The condition is soon reversed as their bodies adjust to the heavier stress of the training.

While it is true that anything can be taken to an unhealthy extreme, it does not happen very often in the case of exercise. The greater risk lies in doing too little, not too much. By way of illustration, ask yourself how many people you have heard of who over-exercise. Now ask yourself how many people you know who do too little exercise. Most of the people I know are sedentary and not at any risk of doing too much. On the other hand, I've never met anyone who does too much.

Because men are subject to some of the diseases thought to be limited to women, I will point out that men also get breast cancer. I will never forget the day that I was talking to Lou P. We had just met and, knowing who I was, he said, "We have more in common than you think!" With that, he whipped open his shirt, exposing a long, horizontal scar, a souvenir from a modified radical mastectomy. So, guys, breast self-exam is for everybody!

With all the hoopla about women getting enough calcium, it may come as a surprise to you to know that men are also subject to osteoporosis. Although they do not suffer the abrupt drop of their sex hormone levels the way women do, the other negative influences of not enough exercise, high protein diets, and the lessening of their hormones all conspire to put men into a negative calcium balance. Luckily for them, men start out with denser bones, which is why they are much older before they start having hip fractures, shortening of stature, and dowager's humps.

I'll throw out a bit of information I find absolutely amazing. Did you know that the human female is the only species that undergoes a menopause? All other female mammals maintain an estrus cycle for the duration of their natural lives. This means that they have ovaries that produce sex hormones and maintain sexual activity all their lives.

A point about women's estrogen levels that you need to be aware of is that it only appears to drop abruptly with the onset of menopause. It was actually assumed that the level of estrogen begins dropping around the age of thirty-five, and many doctors recommend estrogen supplements starting then in order to prevent heart disease and bone loss. However, if women eat a vegan, low-fat diet and get lots of exercise, their risk of heart disease drops and they will maintain their bone mass. Many women actually have very high levels of estrogen, or high enough to suffer the symptoms of estrogen dominance and increase their risk of breast cancer. The last thing they need is more estrogen!

Estrogen and Progesterone

Contrary to common belief, there is a great deal about women's hormones that is not widely known. The important role, for example, of progesterone has only recently been discovered.[2] For years it was thought that estrogen levels were usually too low, and estrogen was, and still frequently is, liberally prescribed to women regardless of their symptoms. Whenever a woman complained of premenstrual symptoms (PMS), she was put on estrogen. In fact, she was probably producing too much estrogen. Fibrocystic breasts, fibroids, heavy bleeding, mood swings, weight gain, and bloating are all symptoms of estrogen dominance. Estrogen exposure has increased radically in just a few generations. It has been estimated that before the Industrial Revolution women had approximately 150 menstrual cycles whereas modern women have 400 cycles.

There has been a major increase in exposure to estrogen due to cycles starting earlier, fewer pregnancies, lower lactation rates, shorter lactation times, and later menopause. This excess exposure leads to all those symptoms mentioned above. What would help these women is a vegan, low-fat diet, regular vigorous exercise, and possibly natural progesterone to balance the estrogen. (Natural progesterone is different from progestin, which is a synthetic progesterone and many, even health professionals, confuse the two.) Since progesterone is only produced when women ovulate, we know that when a woman reaches menopause, she is certainly deficient in progesterone. Fortunately, this can be easily remedied with a plant source of progesterone, usually the Wild Mexican Yam (*Dioscorea*).[3] It is frequently applied in the form of a cream (trans-dermal) because when the hormone goes through the skin, it avoids the first pass through the liver. It's one of the liver's jobs to clear hormones from the blood.

Since breast cancer patients will usually not be given estrogen, its use is academic for many women. By contrast, though, progesterone has been discovered to "normalize" cancerous and other abnormal breast cells subject to excess stimulation by estrogen.[4] Progesterone has been shown to reverse osteoporosis and potentiate your own thyroid hormones. It also maintains a woman's libido.

Female hormones play at least a partial role in many functions of the body, including maintenance of the secondary sex characteristics such as the development of breasts, soft skin, the higher-pitched voice, hair growth rates and patterns, vaginal health, bone strength, healing rates, etc. Your diet, however, significantly influences your level of estrogen, with vegetarian women having lower estrogen levels. Vegetarian women also produce twice the fecal bulk as omnivorous women and excrete more estrogen. Even urinary levels of estrogen are lower in vegetarian women. Since estrogen is easily reabsorbed through the intestinal walls, this leaves less estrogen available for re-absorption and, thus, is another factor in lowering your risk of breast cancer. There are even possible applications of trans-dermal progesterone for men that are beginning to be explored, such as shrinking the prostate and stopping the growth of prostate cancer.

There are so many good reasons for both men and women to take good care of themselves, but probably the most sensual aspect of fitness is the glowing vitality that a fit person exudes. That, to me, is the sexiest of all!

The Fountain of Youth?

Vitality is no respecter of age, and fitness seems to put a hold on the aging process, if not actually reversing it. There are a number of ways to measure the body's biological age. Among them are strength, speed, flexibility, endurance, blood pressure, resting heart rate, body fat percentage, cholesterol level, and the ability to process oxygen. Strenuous exercise along with a low-fat, high complex-carbohydrate diet affects every one of these measures. This, therefore, is the closest thing you'll ever find to a "fountain of youth!"

A sad fact is that as people get older, they tend to put on more body fat even if they don't gain a pound. This is not sexy, right? Bodies that are lean, muscular, and taut are attractive at any age. One way to fight increasing body fat is to exercise. The fun way to exercise is to train. And the way to keep you training is to enter races. Races are also a lot of fun, which is why people keep coming back.

There is also a role that glowing good health plays on the sex drive. When you feel good about yourself and your body, a natural sex appeal just exudes from your pores. You are attractive to other people, and you'll probably find yourself turned on by other sexy, fit bodies. Wouldn't you like to have a healthy, active sex life until you're in your eighties and even nineties?

The old saying "Use it or lose it" definitely applies here. As women age, they experience symptoms of the post-menopausal period such as thinning of the vaginal walls and lack of lubrication. According to some authorities, the best treatment is continued and frequent usage. Gynecologists can usually tell if older women are not sexually active by the thinning and shrinkage of the vagina. In fact, there is one authority that claims that women should remain sexually active all their lives to keep their vaginal tissue healthy, even if they have to do it through masturbation.[5]

Swimming is Sexy!

A study reported in *Swim* Magazine indicated that middle-aged and older men and women with regular swim workouts had sex lives as active as people in their late twenties and early thirties.[6] As long as they maintained their fitness program, their sexual interest and activity did not decline with age. Swimmers in their sixties were as active as others in their forties. And not only were the swimmers more active sexually, they were enjoying it more, according to the rating scale. This makes sense because making love is a physical act where strength, agility, and endurance count. The weak, tired, and out-of-shape person cannot hold up very well or very long. Strong, energetic, and fit lovers can throw themselves enthusiastically into lovemaking and last a lot longer. Yes, fit people of any age make better lovers.

In this country, unfortunately, sexual activity is considered an activity for the young and beautiful. Our role models for physical attractiveness are in their late teens and early twenties, so the idea of the elderly engaging in sexual activity is a foreign idea to most people. And it's foreign to the elderly themselves if they are in poor physical condition and feel badly about their bodies.

The other extreme is that of older people still physically vigorous, with strong, supple bodies, who still feel good about themselves. They will have the energy and desire to continue active sex lives for as long as they want. And being in superb physical condition apparently makes you want to. The apparent reason for this is that the sex drive is dependent on the so-called male sex hormone, testosterone. I say "so-called" because testosterone is present in women as well though in lesser quantities. Studies have shown that physical activity increases levels of testosterone in both men and women and lowers levels of the so-called female hormone, estrogen. Again, I say "so-called" because men also produce estrogen, though likewise in lesser quantities.

This explains why women who train excessively may stop having their menstrual periods. Excessive training in both sexes can have a deleterious effect on the sex drive, probably due to fatigue and a lot less time in their day. These women's sex drive–levels usually return quickly when the over-training stops. This resurgence is probably accelerated by the fact that athletes rated themselves as feeling and looking younger and more attractive than other people their same age.

If You Knew What Alcohol Did To Your Body

Now a word about alcohol and its effects on your body. First of all, you should know that alcohol is toxic to all living cells. Its effects are so scary that if most people knew what it did to their systems, I bet they'd stay as far away from it as possible.

Because alcohol is a solvent, it gets to every cell in your body. It then changes the biochemical functions inside every cell. Because drugs plug into the receptor sites on the surface of the cell membrane, they can cause so-called "desirable" sensations (intoxication). They also cause changes in the bilipid (fat) layers of the cells, although there is less damage if you are on a low-fat diet. Alcohol also causes general havoc in cell receptor function and can even destroy receptors.

Your liver has more than 400 different functions, one of which is to detoxify poisons such as alcohol. Unfortunately, chronic use of alcohol knocks off liver cells. Liver enzymes start leaking into the blood stream. Continued exposure to alcohol leads to hepatitis and cirrhosis (scarring). The liver then contracts, which causes an increase in blood pressure. The poor, besieged liver is then hampered in its function to break down estrogen. Since many alcoholic beverages (primarily beer, sake, and bourbon) contain significant quantities of the plant form of estrogen, (phytoestrogen), this builds up in the body.

If you're a woman, the increase of estrogen heightens your risk of breast cancer. If, however, you're a man, this is really bad news for your sex life. Your testicles will start to shrivel and breasts will start to form. In fact, enlarged breasts (gynecomastia) are a telltale sign that physicians look for in checking for alcoholism. Men become impotent, fertility is impaired, and both men and women suffer loss of libido (sex drive) and become anorgasmic (unable to have an orgasm). If you value your sexuality, you sure have enough reasons to stay away from alcohol.

So, you see, there's a lot more to glowing, good health than most people realize. Fitness is sexy and if you're fit enough to do triathlons you'll probably be in top sexual form as well. Triathlons are sexy for several reasons, and now you know what triathletes are referring to when they talk about the fourth event!

Chapter Sixteen

Beauty Tips for Athletes

One of the more common misconceptions is that women athletes are "jocks" or "jockettes." With that is the implication that being athletic is the antithesis of being feminine—that a "beautiful competitor" is an oxymoron. As I got more and more into hard training and competition, I felt the inevitable conflicts occurring. If I do a swim workout, I'll ruin my hair and I might as well forget about make-up. The same was true of biking and running. Putting a bicycle helmet on my head meant a flattened, sweaty head of hair. And who can present a decent face when you're dripping with perspiration? There was another conflict. On race day you usually have to get up way before the crack of dawn, sometimes 3:00 or 4:00 in the morning. Who could possibly be thinking of looking gorgeous at a time like that, especially when one's mind needs to be on race preparation?

Not being willing to give up all vestiges of attractiveness, I developed a bunch of beauty tricks. Some of them are very practical and some purely frivolous. I would not give up any of them. See if any of these suits you.

Permanent eyeliner and brows. When applied correctly, this make-up technique is done once and forgotten forever. You wake up with beautiful eyes and brows; you come out of the water with beautiful eyes and brows; you cross the finish line with beautiful eyes and brows. I've had mine long enough that I "own" them, feeling they are so much a part of me that I forget I ever really needed them.

In fact, with the liner and brows, I get by without any make-up. This really paid off when the reporters from the *New Zealand Herald* took photos of me right after crossing the finish line of that Ironman. The picture on the front page of that newspaper shows eyes that could have just stepped out of a make-up artist's studio! (Well, almost!)

Dealing with presbyopia. When I reached the age of forty-seven I finally had to face the fact that reading small print was becoming impossible. As I looked around at others approaching forty, they were having to convert to bifocal glasses. I thought that maybe I'd escape that fate, but, no, I was just lucky in being able to put it off longer. When I mentioned to my boss that I was going to have to see an eye doctor, he revealed to me his "secret." He wore contact lenses with one eye set for close-up reading and the other for distance (mono vision).

Since my distance vision was fine, I asked Stan Yamane, my new optometric doctor, if I could wear just one lens. He said he didn't see any reason why I couldn't. I asked if he had any other patients doing that, and he told me I would be the first. Well, this was a little scary, but I figured I didn't have much to lose. And it worked like a charm. For years now, I have been able to avoid eyeglasses and it's been wonderful. I come out of the water able to see everything. If I have a bike problem, I can see close-up details. And, after the race, I can read the race results, and since I frequently cover race events as a reporter, I can start writing the story without having to find eyeglasses.

When the LASIK (Laser-assisted in situ keratomileusis) surgery became available to correct far-sightedness, I made the jump and gave up contact lenses. I now have that eye corrected for reading and have the same results without glasses or contact lenses. The freedom is wonderful. Even more important is to have eyes that stay healthy and functional. This is another case of diet being important. Studies show that those who eat the most green leafy vegetables have the lowest risk of cataracts and glaucoma.[1] Furthermore, this diet prevents age-related macular degeneration—the most common cause of blindness in those over sixty-five.[2]

"Permanent" jewelry. My aunt Dorisse taught me when I was young that it was better to have good jewelry, i.e., the "real" thing. Even if this meant fewer pieces, they should be tasteful and, if need be, expensive. After I lost my earlobes to the plastic surgeon, who made them into nipples as part of my cancer reconstructive surgery, (see Chapter Eighteen), I treated myself to a pair of large, diamond stud earrings.

Now, who wants to keep a treasure like that in a safe deposit box or in a vault? I decided I wanted to wear mine all the time. In order not to risk losing the earrings in the ocean or anywhere else, I bent the posts and put the backs on as usual. Now, they can't come off. Well, I can take them off to clean them, but I don't think I will ever lose them accidentally. I also wear a diamond tennis bracelet with a safety clasp that can't come undone. A good jeweler can solder the fastenings, ensuring they won't be lost. The reason I emphasize "tasteful" is that you will wear them on all occasions. And I for one can't think of an occasion when diamond earrings and bracelets are not nice to have on.

Rings, however, are a problem. I've not found a way to prevent losing them and have just quit wearing them. I do have some gold chains I wear around my neck. If you have the clasps checked at least annually, there is a good chance you will never lose them. Again, I'd rather use them, and take a chance on losing them, than have them sit in a safe deposit box where no one can enjoy them. And, as with the eyeliner and brows, it's nice to come out of the water or cross the finish line looking as feminine and glamorous as I can.

Hair and Skin. I've had it short; I've had it down to my waist. Either way works for me, but short hair is certainly a lot easier to stuff under a swim cap, helmet, or shampoo after the multitudinous workouts we have to undergo. There is probably only one prerequisite, and that is to have a simple hairstyle. And when you exude good health, you don't need to rely on fancy hair-do's to make you beautiful. Then when you cross the finish line of a race, all you have to do is run a comb through your hair. You'll look perfectly groomed, ready for the cameras!

What applies to hair also applies to skin. When your blood is healthy, laden with nutrients, and your circulation top-notch, your skin fairly glows. You don't need any kind of cover-up other than a sun block. Sweat, salt water, chlorine, etc. will not harm your skin. But the sun will.

There is no quicker way to age your skin than with exposure to the sun. Since it's a little difficult to get in your training in the dark, the only solution is to use as close to a total sun block as possible. There are some on the market with a sun protection factor (SPF) of forty-three. This means that, theoretically, you could spend forty-three hours in the sun and get the exposure of one hour. If you're allergic to one of the common ingredients in sun block, PABA, get one with PABA esters, which should eliminate the allergic reactions. The application of a sun block should be an automatic morning ritual, even if you don't plan on a sun workout. It'll pay off as you get older!

Sunglasses. The sun's damage is not limited only to your skin. It could also damage your eyes, causing cataracts to form. Studies have shown that blue-eyed people in the tropics who do not wear sunglasses have a much greater prevalence of cataracts than brown-eyed people who wear sunglasses. Just make sure the lenses are coated with a filter to screen out ultraviolet rays. Sunglasses also tend to minimize the frown lines between the eyes and squinting (laughingly called laugh lines), both of which also lead to wrinkling of the face.

Legs. I'm sure you've seen women, some even quite young, who have disfiguring spider veins or even large, knotty varicose veins in their legs. These are preventable but probably not entirely reversible, although it's probably possible to stop their progression. To prevent them, you need to eat a high-fiber diet like the one described in this book and get lots of large muscle exercise like running and biking.

Varicose veins are caused by failure of the venous valves to stop the backflow of blood as it journeys from the feet up to the heart. As you can imagine, there's a lot of pressure from that blood trying to go upstream, and incompetent valves will let the blood pool in the veins. That pooling leads to tortuous, twisted, knotted veins. Not only is it unattractive, but it can even be fatal as blood clots form in the stagnating blood. It has been said that exercise is the body's second heart.

A lot of people feel that varicose veins are hereditary because they run in families. Well, naturally, the tendency to have the same kind of valves your parents do is inherited. There is nothing, however, you can do about your heredity at this late date, but there is something you can do to improve the health of your veins: Exercise! Are you wondering what a high-fiber diet has to do with varicose veins? People on low-fiber diets have bowel problems like constipation. Constipation causes straining which puts tremendous pressure on the veins in the lower half of the body. Not only will constipated people get varicose veins in their legs, they'll also get hemorrhoids!

Feet. With proper-fitting shoes, or preferably no shoes (nature's way, after all), we should all have beautiful feet. Unfortunately, it doesn't turn out that way. Athletes have black toenails from running downhill in shoes that are too short; blisters from rubbing on areas where there is friction; and thickened toenails from hitting against the ends of shoes with a toe box that is too small. These are usually temporary conditions that are relieved by getting rid of the offending shoes.

Feet expand with usage and most people find their feet grow a size or two when they take up running. Therefore, be sure to get a size large enough to accommodate the spreading foundation for your body. Feet also tend to expand from morning to evening, so buy shoes late in the day. Bike shoes, on the other hand, are fitted differently. They need to be very snug as the body's forces are transmitted through them to the bike pedal, and you will probably need to do little, if any, walking in them. Since most people tend to develop calluses on the bottoms of their feet, take every opportunity you can to walk barefoot in the sand. Not only will this strengthen foot muscles, it will grind off the calluses, leaving baby-smooth skin.

Personally, I think most of the advice given in the so-called "beauty books" is a bunch of garbage, intended only to cater to the dreams of people who want to be more attractive. After all, as I said before, we know now that the high-protein and liquid-protein diets of the past ruined our kidneys and bones. Any low-calorie diet just puts the body into a starvation mode and causes it to add more fat when the deprivation period is over, which, of course, is inevitable. We also know that exercise is the only way to keep a beautiful body and a sexy silhouette throughout your life span. Muscles that don't get used will atrophy and become weak and slack. Sexy curves are from toned muscles, not from silicone or a scalpel. Bones that don't get stressed regularly suffer the same fate of atrophy and weakness.

You don't need make-up to make your skin glow. Your "rouge" is the natural color of the vasomotor flush of strenuous exercise. Your "foundation" is the soft, fine-pored skin that is the result of good nutrients brought to the epithelial cells by a strong circulatory system. Lipstick is unnecessary when lips are healthy and pink from the underlying bright red blood. Teeth look whiter when gums are pinker. And don't forget to floss daily, because all the exercise in the world does not get rid of the plaque that develops around the gum lines which can cause the loss of even healthy teeth. Bright, sexy eyes are the result of an adequate amount of the deep sleep of the physically exhausted, plus the enthusiasm for life and joy of living you feel when the body is treated as it would be if we only came with an "owner's manual."

So, forget about artificial beauty tricks. When in doubt about whether or not to try something, use the following guidance: Is it natural? Now, that doesn't automatically mean if it isn't that you shouldn't do it. It just means you have to know what you are doing and evaluate the risk versus the benefit. All I'm offering here is a way to make lifetime exercise a lot of fun, a very strong habit, and a major commitment. I know that once you try this lifestyle, you'll never go back to the old ways—ever. Just know that when you are your healthiest, you will automatically be at your most beautiful—for the rest of your life!

Chapter Seventeen

Anemia and Accidents:
Why Being Careful Helps

One of the more interesting aspects of my journey to become an Ironman has been the opportunity to learn a lot about my body and human bodies in general. As I increased my training levels in running by doing ultramarathons (any run greater than a marathon, 26.2 miles), I started to notice increasing fatigue. Isn't this normal, you ask? No, not in this case. Besides increasing fatigue, I noticed that after a long, hard run or race I experienced light-headedness. Right after crossing the finish line of my first fifty-kilometer race, I nearly passed out. Knowing enough to get my head down, I headed for the curb of the street and quickly got my head between my knees.

My thoughts at this time were, "Wow, I guess I'm really pushing my limits!" I felt my reaction was normal and of no real concern. When I went to stand up again a few minutes later, however, I nearly passed out again. I started to get a little concerned since it was then close to midnight, and I had to drive myself home.

Somebody brought me some food and drink that I quickly downed, thinking that my blood sugar must be too low. After a few more minutes, I felt much better. I climbed into my car and made it home and went to bed. The next morning when I woke up I still felt light-headed. Furthermore, I discovered I had "melena"—black, tarry stools. This is the hallmark of gastrointestinal (GI) bleeding. I called the emergency room (ER) of the now-very-familiar Tripler Hospital and described the symptoms, asking if this was of any real concern. When they told me, "Get yourself immediately into the hands of competent medical care," I realized it must be serious.

This happened in 1984 when most medical personnel did not know a great deal about some of the maladies that affect long-distance runners. These symptoms could be life-threatening, they emphasized. It was assumed that it was my distance running that was causing my internal bleeding.

One of the first things they did was to try to put a nasogastric (NG) tube into my stomach. Of all the medical procedures I've ever had done, this was by far the most unpleasant. It involved sticking a tube, lubricated by KY jelly, into a nostril, trying to miss the trachea while aiming for the esophagus. You probably know that the trachea leads to the lungs and, if blocked, makes it impossible to breathe—a feeling that causes extreme panic. Well, wouldn't you guess that it was my trachea they hit? With the tube totally blocking the entrance to the trachea, I started gagging and struggling to breathe. With my windpipe totally blocked, I panicked and started to swing wildly. They quickly pulled the tube out and apologized profusely. They said they needed to try again, but I was too shaken.

The experience was so unpleasant that I refused. No amount of pleading was going to change my mind, so they brought in some reinforcements. The chief of the ER said that I could be bleeding to death and that this was the only way to see what was going on.

I told him I was sure I wasn't bleeding to death, and, besides, I had to leave to get to my track workout. The doctor looked aghast!

"You're not going anywhere," he said. "You don't seem to realize the seriousness of the situation. We are going to have to hospitalize you. We have to find the source of the bleeding. Now, I know what you just went through was extremely unpleasant, but we've got more experienced people who will not miss this time."

I was in turmoil. I sat there for a long time trying to reason things out. If these doctors were right, I would need to agree to them trying the procedure again. I thought then about the fainting and melena. Then those panicky feelings would recreate themselves. He let me weigh the pros and cons for a while.

"I will do my best to minimize the discomfort," said the doctor. "We've got to find the source of the bleeding."

I resigned myself to what seemed the inevitable. This time the doctor hit the esophagus and fed the tube into the stomach. Attaching a syringe to the end of the tube, he started aspirating the contents of my stomach. In spite of the discomfort of a tube through my nose and down my throat and into my stomach, I watched wide-eyed, intrigued by what was going on. What was coming out of my stomach looked like coffee grounds.

"Uh-oh," said the medical staff. "That's bad news. You're bleeding from the stomach. There'll be no track workout today. We're keeping you right here!"

Instead of my life passing before my eyes, a vision of my next races, the Boston Marathon and the next Ironman, went flying by. When the results of my blood tests came back from the lab, I was told that I was extremely anemic. My hemoglobin was 6.8; hematocrit twenty-four; my Total Iron-Binding Capacity (TIBC) was 399; and my serum ferritin was six. According to the doctor, what all this meant was that I should be flat on my back getting a blood transfusion. (See Appendix One for an explanation of the laboratory tests.) The situation was serious. I was supposed to be getting on a plane in two days to do the Boston Marathon. All serious runners know that Boston is the Holy Grail of runners. I had worked too hard to qualify for Boston and was not giving it up.

I begged and I pleaded. "Look," I said. "I just finished a fifty-kilometer run. If I were in as bad shape as you say, I wouldn't have been able to do that."

The doctor shook his head. "I don't know how you did it, but you are risking damage to your heart muscle by insisting on doing this. Being this anemic, your blood can't carry enough oxygen to support the demands of a marathon on your heart. You're crazy to even consider it."

I felt convinced. After all, I was doing this for fitness and to beat cancer, so it didn't make sense to create damage to my heart while trying to get stronger. I skipped the track workout, and spent the night in the "Tripler Hotel."

The next day I was "scoped." This means that an endoscope was passed into my stomach and upper intestine to let the doctors see what condition my GI tract was in. To my surprise and delight, everything appeared normal. As I questioned how this could be, I was told that the lining of the GI tract heals very rapidly, sometimes in fewer than twenty-four hours. They even showed me Polaroid photos of my insides. Yep, completely healed.

A devious thought crept into my head. "Do it!" it said.

I dismissed it.

"Yes, you can," it said again.

Hmmmm, I can always stop anytime during the race, I thought. Yes! That's it! I'm going to Boston, and I will at least, I told myself, start the race. Armed with a load of iron pills, I arrived at the start of one of the most prestigious races in the world, thrilled at even being there. I ran the race slowly and carefully, monitoring my body signals all the way. The only real symptom I noticed was that I was cold. Since the temperature was in the low thirties, I didn't think too much about it and just put on the gloves I'd brought and wrapped myself in a plastic garbage bag that some kind, anonymous soul gave me.

My racing singlet read "Hawaii" across the front but, of course, was not visible through the bag. I figured that after a few miles, when I'd warmed up, I'd take the garbage bag off. After all, I was pretty proud of being all the way from Hawaii and knew I would probably get a lot of attention from the spectators who line the marathon course. I also knew I was going to need the interaction and encouragement from the spectators to help me get through the 26.2 miles I was facing in this apparently weakened condition.

At the ten-mile mark, I took off the gloves. Within minutes, my fingers got so numb I couldn't hold the paper cups supplying liquid refreshment at the aid stations. I knew I needed to drink a lot of water. On went the gloves again. At the twenty-mile mark, I was still cold. This is ridiculous, I thought. But, what the heck, since I was that cold, I figured I had better keep the garbage bag on. In retrospect, I think it was the anemia that kept me from warming up.

Then I saw the official photographer taking pictures of all the runners. Enough's enough, I thought, and off came the garbage bag. I was not about to have my official photo showing me doing the Boston Marathon in a garbage bag. I finished Boston in a decent time and was glad I'd persisted, gambled, and won. What an experience and an exciting race to do! It took months of iron pills to get me back to normal. First, my hemoglobin came back up to normal over a period of about three months, but it was nearly a year before my iron stores registered normal.

The main lesson I learned was to monitor the color of my stools. Any bleeding from the GI tract causes darker stools and is immediately obvious when you're a vegetarian. A plant-based diet yields light-colored stools, whereas animal products (digested blood) yield dark stools. I have learned that running hard races and triathlons may cause several days of GI bleeding. I don't yet know how to prevent this and, consequently, have frequent hemoglobin checks. Reading medical journals, I know that this bleeding is common in long-distance runners.

Most physicians I have talked to seem to think that the bleeding comes from the stomach, but Kent C. Holtzmuller, M.D. claims that the bleeding comes from the colon.[1] He explains that the stomach has a double blood supply and is not as vulnerable to the effects of blood being shifted to the working muscles. But the colon, he claims, has only a single blood supply and, as a result, suffers damage due to the lack of blood to the cells, which then die. He also states that almost all marathoners have traces of blood in their stools at the end of a race.

I also found out the hard way that non-steroidal anti-inflammatory medications cause the same thing: GI bleeding. Over a period of ten years I've found that there are no anti-inflammatories that will not cause me GI bleeding. As a result, I wonder how many people have GI bleeding and don't know it. If you eat the typical American diet filled with animal products, you'd have to bleed quite a lot to see black, tarry stools. It's surprising how little physical activity it really takes to cause some bleeding. There is a test for occult bleeding that you might be able to get from your doctor to check at home. I do this test routinely, not just for GI bleeding from racing but as a check for colon cancer. The American Cancer Society recommends this test annually for patients over forty or fifty years of age.

The Crash I Can't Remember: Safety Comes First!

As if all the other medical problems I'd had to contend with in the lead-up to my first Ironman weren't enough, I had a bike crash that laid me up for six weeks. Since it happened only seven weeks before the Ironman, things looked pretty grim for my getting to the start line.

Preparation for any race involves knowing the course. Since the Ironman bike course was on the Big Island of Hawaii, I'd gone to the Island seven weeks before to practice the swim, bike, and run. My father had all sorts of misgivings about my riding a bike on these roads in Hawaii, feeling they were fraught with danger. It wasn't as if I felt otherwise; it was that I was willing to take the risk. Although by no means an expert cyclist, I did feel I took no unreasonable risks.

In late August 1984, I was tooling along the Queen Kaahumanu Highway at about mile ninety-seven of the 112-mile course. I was just a few miles from the village of Kona. The last thing I remember is passing the turn-off to the airport, thinking how good I felt and confident I was going to be able to do the bike leg with no problems.

The next thing I remembered was that it was 10:30 p.m. and I was in a hospital bed, feeling pain literally from head to toe.

I asked the nurse what happened and where my bike was.

"We told you," she laughed. "Don't you remember?"

A medical technologist came in to draw some blood and started talking to me as if she knew me. I was totally confused! She laughed and said, "You've asked me at least a dozen times already, 'What happened and where is my bike?' "

"I asked you?" I said incredulously.

"Yeah," she said, "when I drew your blood this afternoon. You asked everybody in sight."

"But hospital personnel wouldn't know things like where my bike was," I replied.

"Well, you asked them anyway," she said. "Then when they told you, two minutes later you asked them again, and again!"

Boy, was my mind reeling from the shock. Here I was, in a hospital, not knowing how I got there, and people were telling me things I didn't even remember saying. Slowly, I was able to piece the story together. A passing pick-up truck had apparently grazed me and knocked me off my bike. I was found unconscious by the side of the road. A motorist who witnessed the crash called an ambulance with his CB radio. The ambulance crew checked vital signs and determined that I had suffered concussion, that I was not in need of an IV, that I had suffered some kind of impact fall, and that I was going to require the services of an emergency room.

Luckily, I had a helmet on. No, I shouldn't say "luckily." I had learned from my very first days of cycling that a helmet was an absolute necessity when riding and, therefore, wouldn't even go around the block without one. In any case, I hit the ground hard enough to crack the helmet open and sustain a three-inch long cut on the side of my head. In fact, I was handed my helmet in two halves. The doctors said that if I hadn't been wearing it, I would probably have been killed. My feet had been tightly strapped to the pedals by metal toe clips. The metal straps had been sheared off.

Now, in a hospital bed, I tried to move. The stabbing pain in my hip brought me up short. "Oh, my God, what happened to me?" I wailed, on the verge of tears. The medical personnel tried to reassure me that I was going to be all right.

"I've got an Ironman in seven weeks!" I said.

They shook their heads. "No way!" they said.

The doctor shook his head, too. "No way! Look, just forget it for this year. Get well, and plan for it next year."

But I had my own thoughts about what I was going to do. I'd invested too much in this venture. I felt that if breast cancer couldn't stop me, I wasn't about to let anything else keep me from doing the Ironman.

I wanted to get out of that bed and get back to my training routine. I felt just like I did after my cancer surgeries. The plotting and scheming started immediately, primarily because I didn't want my conditioning to go down the tubes! All I could think about was getting out of there. I wanted to get back to my running, swimming, and, yes, biking.

More than anything else, what bothered me was the amnesia. I could remember passing the airport road, but I had been found two miles past it. I couldn't remember being hit, or any of the people who had stopped to help me. I couldn't remember the ambulance ride, the emergency room repairs consisting of stitching up the gash in my head, the x-rays, the blood-drawing, all the bandages covering what they said was a "seven-point landing," and who knows what else. Then there was also the fact that my brain seemed to be short-circuiting: "What happened? Where's my bike?"

The nurses seemed amused by the whole situation, but I was really upset. Why couldn't I remember? The doctor on call at the time was Frank Ferren, M.D., who was himself an Ironman athlete and who had, as it turned out, treated a number of bike crash victims. He explained that what I had was anterograde and retrograde amnesia; that is, after a concussion, people sometimes forget things that happened immediately prior to the impact as well as after.

As I was in the hospital for almost a week, I spent hours mentally digging through my brain cells. "Remember, darn it, remember!" It was months later, when I was still mentally digging, that all of a sudden I remembered sharp, needle-like pains. That was the stitching up the cut in my head. Then I recalled a vague image of an elevator. Yes, that was a ride on a gurney to my hospital room. Then I remembered three or four people trying to move me off the gurney. I obviously had not been sedated; I had screamed in pain as they lifted me up onto the bed.

The hip pain was no better a week later. When I went to see an orthopedic specialist back in Honolulu, the doctor ordered a bone scan. This test, which involves injecting a radioactive substance into the blood that over the period of a couple of hours settles into areas of bone injury, disclosed a hip fracture.

Not only was my first Ironman at risk, but I'd entered the Waikiki Roughwater Swim which was to take place that weekend. This was important to me because it represented the first event of the Ironman. If I couldn't do this event, I really was in trouble. I had never really given up the idea that, no matter what, I was going to be there for the start of the Ironman.

The orthopedic specialist had the bone scan on the lighted screen. Shaking his head, he said, "No, there's definitely a fracture there. It's going to be six to eight weeks on crutches. Forget the Ironman."

Almost in desperation, I said, "What about swimming? Swimming should be good for it, shouldn't it?"

Looking at me as if I'd lost my marbles, he almost pleaded, "Look, let those bones knit! If you keep moving them, you're taking a chance on permanent damage to your hip. There's a risk of necrosis! Necrosis—death of the bone!"

Now I really *was* in trouble. How could I tell the doctor I'd been swimming daily since getting out of the hospital? He didn't look as if he'd understand if I told him how careful I was about keeping the hip immobile and that I was not kicking my feet and legs at all. Thoroughly frightened and chastened, I gave up. They're right, I thought. Forget it.

That lasted until I got home. I guess the fear wore off, and I found myself scheming and trying to decide how at least to start the Roughwater Swim. Because there were course marshals on surfboards all along the 2.4 mile course, I could drop out at any time.

All that was left to do was to get somebody to take the crutches from me after I got in the water, get them down to the finish line 2.4 miles away, and wade into the water with them so I could walk up the beach to the swim finish line. People thought I was crazy to even think of it but finally agreed when they saw I was determined to swim in that race with or without their help.

And, so it was, in 1984, that I learned that swimming for a triathlete is primarily an upper body sport. I found that my time was not that much slower, that my dragging legs still acted as a rudder, and that I could do things I "shouldn't" if I wanted to badly enough.

Now, this is not to say that the doctors were wrong. The safest course, surely, is to rest after an injury. It's just that you're taking a chance if you persist in training in the face of an injury. I was really lucky, and, in fact, healed much faster than the medical estimates indicated I would. I was off the crutches in four weeks instead of the six to eight weeks predicted. Based on the experience of a whole lot of injuries and seven surgeries, I have seen that the fit athlete heals much faster than the average, sedentary person.

Healing Fast

The rest of the recovery proceeded at an accelerated pace. After the Roughwater Swim, I started toying with the idea of getting on a stationary bicycle. I argued with myself for another week, and thought, what the heck, if it hurts, I'll just stop. Sure enough, after just a couple of minutes, it did. I did not persist. I wasn't really disappointed or depressed either, though, thinking that I'd just keep trying until the day it was all right. And I'd know exactly when that day was. The next morning I was thinking that I'd had another twenty-four hours of healing time. Time to try again!

To my surprise, I could go four minutes before pain set in. On the third day, the time doubled again. I got very excited as I computed the recovery rate. Now I already knew I had the swim handled; here it looked as though the bike leg was going to be okay, too. Sure enough, each day I saw this tremendous rate of improvement. Ironically, I was also entered in the *Honolulu Advertiser* "Century Ride"—about five weeks after the accident. Here was my chance to see if could do a 100-miler on the bike. To my greatest surprise and delight, I made it through the entire 100 miles without too much pain. I knew it then! I was going to do at least the first two parts of the Ironman for sure.

On the medical check-up scheduled five weeks after the crash, I told the doctor that I thought I was really healing ahead of schedule. He poked, prodded, and apparently was satisfied that I was not going to yell out in pain.

He backed away, putting his hands on his hips. "Let's see if you can walk," he said. After one week in the hospital and four weeks on crutches, I almost panicked.

"Walk?" I said.

I suddenly got cold feet. I'd grown attached to those crutches and was not sure I was ready for the real showdown. What if I couldn't walk? The Ironman was now only two weeks away. I slowly, carefully put some weight on my right foot. It seemed okay. I put on a little more weight. Still okay. The doctor held out a steadying hand, and I put the rest of the weight on my foot.

"Ohmygod!" I whooped. I was standing and nothing hurt! Another slow series of weight transfers, this time to the left foot. And, ohmygod, no pain! Another step, and another. I let the joy sink in, "I'm okay... I'm okay!"

"All right, now, just take it easy," the doctor said. "You've still got a ways to go, Don't get exuberant and do too much."

The next day I ran for two minutes and was about to discover that getting back to running was just like getting back to biking, except that the Ironman was now only thirteen days away and I was going to have to run a full marathon. I couldn't keep doubling my time, so I stopped a week before the race with a single twelve-mile run. At that point I didn't care what happened, because however it worked out, I would be there at the start line and would go as far as I could.

As it turned out, I had a wonderful first Ironman. Because of all that had occurred the previous seven weeks, survival was all that was on my mind. There was not even the slightest wish to "race." That, as it turned out, was the best thing that could have happened to me. It forced me to pace myself and, as a result, I finished in fourteen hours forty-nine minutes.

The official results weren't available until the next morning. When I saw that I was one minute from placing in my age group, I was so excited that I immediately started plotting my training schedule. Just think what I could do if I could train for the last seven weeks, I mused. Just wait until next year! On top of that, I was going to be in a new age group, the fifty to fifty-four year olds. It would help being the youngest in my group instead of what I had been, the oldest.

Now, if could only remember that ambulance ride!

Chapter Eighteen

Reconstructing a Body and a Life

Amid those harrowing days of dealing with the diagno-sis of cancer and getting ready for the mastectomy, there appeared a small ray of sunshine. I'd remembered reading about reconstructive surgery and asked my surgeon about it. He said he'd arrange to have a consultation with the Plastic Surgery Department.

One of the books I'd read said that there was a "quaint" theory that still existed in the minds of some plastic surgeons regarding breast reconstruction. They were recommending that breast reconstruction be withheld from women for approximately two years. It was felt that if a woman had to do without for at least that period of time, when the reconstruction was accomplished she'd be grateful for whatever she got. It seems the technology was not that great, and, in fact, some of the least successful results bordered on the grotesque.

I had expected to see the plastic surgeon before my mastectomy, but he was "too busy." This dismayed me because another book had suggested that the plastic surgeon should participate in the mastectomy surgical procedure itself to ensure that nothing was done to complicate the later surgery. I had no choice then but to take my chances. As it turned out, there was a good reason for the plastic surgeon to be there.

When I finally saw the plastic surgeon about two months later, he looked at the location of the two drainage tube scars that had been put almost in the middle of where a new breast would be constructed. He shook his head and said that it was too bad they were placed there; the resultant scar tissue had made his job a little harder. I saw nothing to gain by protesting and just heaved a big sigh. There was, however, a change in the surgical procedure between the first and second mastectomies. The second surgical procedure had the scars toward my back, completely away from the reconstructive site. I felt gratified, at least, to see some progress being made, but wondered how many other women, their surgeons, and plastic surgeons had yet to go through this same learning curve. Actually, in some cases today, surgeons will even do a simultaneous mastectomy and reconstruction. I've visited a couple of these patients and have been amazed that they have no idea of how lucky they are. One patient thought that every breast cancer patient was treated this way.

At the time of my first visit to the plastic surgeon, he examined me and told me that I was an excellent candidate for reconstruction. I was elated and asked how soon I could have the operation.

"As soon as the scar softens, and the skin stretches enough to take the implant," he said.

In an effort to get any possible vagrant cancer cells lying under the skin and in the subcutaneous fat, surgeons cut away as much skin as possible and scrape the subcutaneous fat from the "flaps" they create to cover the now-bare chest and close the wound. The resulting upper torso now looks flatter than a prepubertal child's. The ribs stick out, and it's difficult to move the arms in any direction due to the skin having been stretched tightly to cover the chest wall.

The plastic surgeon told me that it would take a minimum of six months to a year for the scar to soften and the skin to stretch. Indeed, it might never happen. This is when they do skin grafts, a prospect I did not relish at all. I very conscientiously did stretching exercises and even pulled on the skin for good measure. It must have worked because during my third visit at four months the surgeon told me that I had made progress. We planned my surgery for two months later.

Looking back, I don't know how I got through those days. Every shower, every swim, every glance in the mirror was a stark reminder of not only a breast-less form but also of the cancer. Stuffing bras with a prosthesis just did not do the trick. Every time I raised my arm, the whole bra slid up. When I lowered my arm, the bra and prosthesis stayed up. What an uncomfortable, miserable way to live! I felt like I was holding my breath until the day of the surgery.

The day I was admitted to hospital, I had to go through all the usual pre-op tests. This time, in contrast to the previous occasions, I did so with great joy and cheer. I grinned at the lab techs as they drew my blood. I babbled on as the electrocardiogram technician checked the condition of my heart, saying that this was the last time that electrodes were going to be placed on this chicken-breasted form. She paid no attention to me as she seemed to be having trouble with the machine. I asked if something was wrong. She then turned to me, saying, "Are you a *runner*?"

"Yes, why?" I asked.

"That explains it," she said. "I was getting a heart rate of 44!" Since the average adult heart rate is about 72, this put me in the extremely fit category, and she had never seen a woman with a heart rate that low.

The plastic surgeon then took his purple marker and drew all sorts of marks on me. He drew a nipple line across the chest so that the nipples would be even, two circles for the areolas (the pigmented areas around the nipples), two lower lines for the inframammary fold (medical talk for the lower curves of my new breasts), and marks on my ears and thighs.

My earlobes were going to contribute a wedge of skin that was to be sculpted into two nipples, and my upper inner thighs were to contribute the skin for two new areolas.

"Just the right hint of pink, too," the plastic surgeon joked.

That night in the hospital I could hardly sleep. The plastic surgeon had impressed on me that the choices I had made as to the exact size and location of my new breasts were irreversible. I'd better be sure, he said. I got up several times during the night to check myself in the mirror. Were they going to be too big? Too small? Too high? Too low? Too far apart? Too close together?

My God, I thought. What did they used to look like? I couldn't remember! I thought then that maybe some of those surgeons had the right idea—make them wait and they'll be grateful for anything. And I was, for a while. The healing seemed to go very well for the first month, but one day I noticed that one "breast" was a little high. Or was it that the other one was too low? Over the period of a couple of months, one or the other was happening. I returned for a check-up and remarked on the discrepancy.

The plastic surgeon brushed off my concern, saying that nothing on our bodies that is paired is identical, that our feet are two different sizes, our legs are two different lengths, and so on. I told him that while I agreed to a point, this had passed that point! I felt like a ship whose cargo had shifted and was "listing" to one side. Finally, when he realized I was not going to be mollified, he agreed to do the correction.

By this time I was an old hand at surgery, and the thought of another operation didn't bother me in the least. It is a process, much like a marathon. You've got to go through a lot of discomfort sometimes to get what you want, and, like a marathon, it's worth it in the end. Today, the whole process has been somewhat reversed. My new breasts are so much a part of me and my body image that I've forgotten what I used to look like. And the best news of all is that as I grow older, they will never sag. I sometimes chuckle to myself as I conjure up the image of a ninety-year-old triathlete with these two nice, high, firm, round bosoms!

Chapter Nineteen

Ironman: Kona, Hawaii

The tiny village of Kona on the Big Island of Hawaii gets transformed every October as the Ironman competitors start arriving. The air is absolutely electric with the tension and deadly seriousness of so many of the triathletes. Alii Drive connects the swim start and finish, the bike start with the bike finish and run start, and for the finale the finish for the marathon. For the six miles in between, there are throngs of people and parked cars along the roadside offering their local, homemade version of support and whatever kind of aid is necessary and legal. But that's where all the help ends.

From Kona to Hawi, fifty-six desolate, deserted, hot, black, lava-covered miles lie in wait for the poor unsuspecting cyclists. And once out of the village for the third event, the by-now exhausted runners have to traverse that same desolation for the ten miles past the airport to the marathon turnaround. There is nothing but deadly heat and boredom. The tedious mile after mile seems to just suck the energy, body fluids, and goals right out of the most committed of competitors.

These are the thoughts that were going through my mind all week long just before my sixth Ironman. I felt strong enough to continue hard training, but the word among all the triathletes was "taper." To taper means to ease off on all those hard miles of training so that the body can recover its energy and strength.

The most common mistake triathletes make is to go into a race tired. It is also very difficult to taper when you've got so much energy. You just can't sit still. We all say we'll start our taper. Then we end up taking "just a short swim to loosen up the shoulders," or "just a short cycle to loosen up the legs," or "just a short run to get rid of some excess energy," and, of course, once started, it's like taking "just one potato chip." It can't be done!

Thou Shalt Know the Course

There were people swimming the evening before the race as well as those who arrived so late that they had no choice but to check things out—the swim, bike, and/or run—at practically the last minute. One of the cardinal rules of racing is, "Know the course."

This is especially true of the Kona Ironman, particularly when there are competitors arriving from all over the world, many of whom have never even been to America, much less Kona, Hawaii. This obviously presents quite a problem when the course covers over forty miles, to say nothing of the frequently extreme conditions. One year, the winds were so strong that they literally blew cyclists off their bikes. The ocean can be so rough that swimmers get too seasick to continue, as their vomiting sucks the strength right out of their bodies. If you're a runner, you know what 114 degrees Fahrenheit can do to you. Needless to say, newly arrived competitors are anxious about the course. You cannot even check out the course in the cool of the evening without grave risk since there aren't any streetlights. The dates of the Ironman are, in fact, selected on the basis of the lunar calendar, and the athletes have until midnight to finish. The light of a full moon is all there is to guide many of the competitors on their quest for the final finish line.

I had feelings of nervousness and anxiety constantly welling up in me. In spite of continuously reminding myself that I had done this several times before and could, therefore, do it again I still felt very apprehensive. I almost envied those who were doing it for the first time; they, after all, did not yet know how bad it could get out there. I also knew that, on each of the five previous Ironman events, I had been on the better side of the odds, and that one of these days, those odds were going to catch up with me.

Some of the fears centered on mechanical problems with the bike. I ride racing wheels with twelve spokes in front and eighteen on the rear. (The usual number of spokes is thirty-six.) This concession to aerodynamics and weight does not inspire confidence in me or anyone who looks at these wheels, usually with great amazement. "Those wheels don't look like they could hold you up," or "You've got more guts than I do, lady," these skeptics say. I have been assured, however, that they are as strong, if not stronger, than the conventionally thirty-six-spoked wheel. And, so far, they've served me well. Five Ironman triathlons without a mishap or even getting out of true!

There was an incident in one of the races when I thought I had a problem. I was coming down the home stretch of the bicycle leg, concentrating only on keeping up my speed. All of a sudden there was a "tick…tick…tick…" with each revolution of my front wheel. I was near panic. Expecting the wheel to collapse at any moment, I put on my brakes, trying to slow down so that when I fell I wouldn't hit the pavement so hard. Then I thought of stopping to try to fix the problem. All the insecurities I've ever had about my limited mechanical prowess came surging at me, and I took the cowardly way out. I kept pedaling. The "tick…tick…tick…" continued unabated but nothing else was happening. With my heart in my throat, I decided to get as close to the bike finish line as possible so as to cut down the distance I would have to carry my bike to the bike transition point. (Triathlon rules say only that you and your bike have to finish; you don't have to be on it. You can carry it!)

By this time my legs were rubbery and shaking as the panic-induced adrenaline was wearing off. I was, to say the least, a nervous wreck. But still nothing was happening. The wheels were still turning and I was still upright on the bike. By this time the finish was in sight. I put on an extra surge of speed, crossed the finish line, dropped the bike, and took off running. It was only on completion of the run that I found out what had happened. The sensor of my speedometer had loosened its attachment to the spoke and was dangling uselessly, hitting the brake with every revolution of the wheel. You can bet that I now frequently check for loose screws on the connector for that errant sensor!

Then there are all the things that can go wrong during the marathon leg. Every time I consider 26.2 miles alone, much less after a 2.4-mile swim and 112 miles of cycling, I still shake my head in disbelief. Logically, it seems to me, it can't be done, especially after some of my 100-mile training rides and the 112-mile Around Oahu Bike Race, when I can barely limp into the finish area.

What this has taught me is that we do what we have to do, and if I program my mind, it will generally (I stress *generally*) keep the body going until the end—whenever that end comes. This is how I cope with differing external and internal conditions. What I see is what I get, and I just get on with it. This plan is not always foolproof as I am reminded periodically when I see one of the burned-out competitors staggering zombie-like in directions not always leading directly to the finish line.

What's even more heart-rending is to see a fallen athlete. It brings tears to my eyes as I wonder why and how our minds can push our bodies up to and even beyond their physical limits. What a demonstration of the power of the mind with its ability to set goals, to visualize their attainment, and the ability to perform what must be self-hypnosis. I still marvel at the genius of this species. We're all pretty incredible when you stop to think about it.

The Sleep of the Exhausted

One thing about heavy training that a lot of athletes notice is that although the anxiety may be pretty devastating we can usually sleep very well. No matter how nervous I've been about these ultra-distance events, I've usually gotten a good night's sleep the night before. After all, sometimes I can hardly hold my eyes open past 10:00 p.m. When I'm really nervous, I tend to wake up very early.

Since most races start at very early hours, it all works out very well. With this much physical activity, you tend to sleep very soundly and it seems that you require less sleep. In fact, I feel that all the body's systems seem to work better with a heavy load of exercise and a good diet.

As it turns out, all these insecurities that come flooding up during the week preceding the Ironman serve a very useful purpose. One should never undertake an event like this lightly, no matter how many times you've done it. Even if your conditioning is as good or better than in past events, there are always different conditions on the course. While it's true that the experience you've gained helps, no two events are ever identical. Nor are you ever exposed to all the risky situations that could ever come up.

Life is not Always Fair

Two weeks before the 1987 Kona Ironman, a competitor was hit by a concrete truck and killed. I knew Pat Griskus, having ridden alongside him in the 1986 Ironman when we were both trying to buoy each other's resolve to keep going at the eighty-mile mark of the bike leg. Pat had lost a leg in a motorcycle accident some years prior. He had gotten an artificial leg, put running shoes on, and was out doing the Ironman. Surely, I thought, if Pat can make it, so must I. It was tragic that he did not make it after all he'd been through.

Riding out in the middle of the lava fields at temperatures over 100 degrees Fahrenheit, I was experiencing a terrible low. I wanted to get off that bike in the worst way and go stretch out on the lava. Reminding myself that the rough lava was no place to lie down, I negotiated with myself to try to keep going until I reached the next aid station. Then, I reasoned, I could lie down where they would have medical aid if I needed it. But the lava kept enticing me. It was not soft, fluffy, cushy, chocolate marshmallow (it was hard, hot, black molten rock). My God, I thought, I must be hallucinating!

Checking the speedometer, I calculated that the next aid station was only a couple of miles away. Surely I could make it to that point, I thought, and then I could lie down. Then I started wondering why I was going through this. It had never happened before. Maybe people were right—three and four Ironman Triathlons in a year are too much for anybody's body. Then I recalled that I had not eaten any food, relying instead on liquid supplements that were supposed to provide you with calories, electrolytes, and fluids.

When I finally made it to the next aid station, I gobbled up everything in sight: bananas, oranges, cookies, and I can't remember what else. Within a few minutes, I could feel the energy coursing through my body. I now felt as if I could make it to the next aid station before lying down. I thought then that I would be able to at least finish the bike leg before lying down. Then, when I finally got to the end of the bike leg, I thought I could at least run a couple of miles to make it a "complete" training day, and then I'd lie down.

After a few miles I realized I was feeling strong enough to run the entire marathon. I could not believe how I'd gone from the extreme of wanting desperately to lie down on that bed of hot lava to completing a marathon and crossing the finish line, feeling so fantastic that I babbled euphorically for three hours after.

That was the memory I had of Pat. He and I shared our feelings about questioning our sanity at even being out there, doing these painful things to our bodies. The shock hit hard as I stared in disbelief at the newspaper article announcing his death. Then I realized that this was not the first time this had happened, and that it could happen to any one of us at any time.

Are we crazy to put ourselves at such high exposure to risk? Are we playing

Russian roulette with our lives? Well, what are the odds? If 1,500 people are competitors and one gets killed, is this a reason to back out of the competition? Is not daily living a risk of one degree or another? Where do we put ourselves on the "risk continuum"? I suppose the least amount of risk exposure is in our own bedroom (certainly not the kitchen or the bathroom). Does it make any sense to say, then, that we should spend our whole lives in our bedroom? Obviously not. Then there's the other extreme of placing ourselves in constant danger. And I guess that's where the answer lies. We each have to determine how much risk we are willing to take in our lives. Without risk there can be no gain; we have to put ourselves on the starting line first.

It's a fact of life that people are more frequently sorry for what they did not do than anything they ever did. So, while I'm not saying everybody should get out there and ride bicycles on the highway or do an Ironman, I am saying that whenever I've taken a risk, I've usually been glad I did.

Being diagnosed with breast cancer has made me even more of a risk-taker. For one thing I've often felt that I had nothing to lose; I was going to die anyway. And, of course, that's true. We will all die anyway. The only thing that's in question is when and how. In my case, I know the probable "how" but not the "when." So my approach changed with the diagnosis of cancer. It made me a lot gutsier. If I'm going to go, I'm going to have done something first.

Nearly Twenty Years Out

Coming up now on nearly twenty years since the diagnosis, my mind conjures up two very contrasting images. One projects ahead thirty years with no recurrence of cancer. I feel sad that I've wasted all that time worrying over all those doctor's visits and tests, with the specter of cancer shadowing everything I've done. Then my mind goes to the immediate future. Maybe tomorrow will be the day the hospital calls to say that the tests show that the cancer has spread in my body and that it is time to start some chemotherapy or radiation, or whatever. If this happens, I would feel the despair of losing those good feelings of invulnerability that have slowly been re-forming in my mind as I get further away from the day of that deadly diagnosis. So which is it to be? This says a lot for living in the present moment, doesn't it? We must make each day count because that really is all any of us has.

A lot of these thoughts come up when I'm doing a long race. There are times when the present moment is extremely uncomfortable, and I wonder why I'm putting myself through this. These are the questions people ask when they are in any stage of life where there is discomfort. The Ironman is a symbolic representation of life, a microcosm of a lifetime. There are the highs and lows in between the start and finish of an event, but there's nothing like getting the reward at the end. This is different for each one of us.

For me each time I have crossed that finish line, I have felt a joy and ecstasy that immediately cancels all the discomfort I'd felt just moments before. Then I get to go around and see those who came in before me, sharing their joy. Next, I get to see those coming in after me and share their moments of finishing an incredible race. The value of doing something like an Ironman or any of my other races usually is emphasized to me when I realize that my usual response after a short recovery period is "Just wait 'til next time!" And every "next time" has just gotten better and better. I wish it never had to end.

Chapter Twenty

What's the Prognosis:
Why Cancer Isn't Curable

ancer is a very scary disease. Even with the advent of AIDS, it is considered the disease people fear the most. "Cancer" usu-ally conjures up an image of a patient ravaged by chemotherapy and radiation who then dies anyway.

Newspapers and magazines regularly report "breakthroughs" in cancer treatments, but the sad fact is that studies of the most common cancers (colon, lung, breast, and prostate) have not been showing longer survival times. For one thing, by the time the cancer is detectable by the usual clinical methods, the tumor has shed the cancer cells and spread throughout the body. Once these cells break off from the primary tumor and are transported to other parts of the body through the circulatory system, it's almost impossible to detect the new colonies until they, too, are large enough to be picked up by blood tests, x-rays, scans, etc. For chemotherapy and radiation to kill all of the cancer cells, the doses have to be so high they nearly kill the patient. These treatments can do irreversible damage to the patient's immune system, and this, after all, is what is keeping us alive. Without it, we are prey to every little bug that comes along.

Another important factor to consider is that improved diagnostic methods mainly mean the patient just finds out about his disease sooner. This artificially lengthens the "survival" time. The natural course of the disease in most cases is still, unfortunately, the same.

What's confusing to a lot of people is how cancer kills. Right after my diagnosis, a few people commented, "Well, it's just a breast." It's not usually the primary, or first, tumor discovered that is fatal, especially in breast, colon, prostate, and skin cancers. It's the metastasis, or spread, of these cells, which break off and set up housekeeping in the liver, bones, lungs, and brain. It's a lot like letting all the horses out of the barn. Tracking them down is extremely difficult, and shooting them down with chemicals and radiation is not only difficult, it's also extremely hazardous to normal cells. That's why chemotherapy and radiation treatments cause nausea, vomiting, and hair loss. The normal cells most vulnerable to these weapons are the fastest growing cells, the lining of our gastrointestinal system and hair. And if it's not powerful enough to cause those side effects, it's not likely to stop the cancer cells, either.

Because oncologists, or cancer specialists, are seeing so little change in the longevity of these patients with the most common kinds of cancer, many are starting to emphasize prevention. Through epidemiological (population) studies, it is very clear that individual countries have their own patterns of frequency of the different kinds of cancers. When many of these frequencies are correlated with dietary differences, a telling pattern emerges.

This is why so many researchers are convinced that colon, breast, and prostate cancers are related to diet. There are almost perfect correlations between frequency of deaths from breast cancer and percentage of dietary fat, according to the findings of K. Carroll, a researcher who published his findings in 1975.[1]

In 1977, A. Lowenthals published a study showing that breast and colon cancers rise together in fifty-six countries of the world.[2] When you look at the similarity in the rising and falling of the cancer rates and the dietary fat, it is striking that nearly all of the variance is explained. In other words, there isn't "room" left for other variables such as genetics, stress, or other environmental factors.

Nature's Experiment

So, while we cannot do the live human experiments we would need to "prove" this theory, we can take advantage of this natural experiment provided us with if we are smart enough to look at the data before us. The few countries that have a greater fat intake than we in the U.S.—the Netherlands, Denmark, New Zealand, for example—also have a greater death rate from breast cancer.

As early as 1963, Ernst Wynder, M.D., and President and founder of the American Health Foundation, noted the fact that Japanese women in Japan with breast cancer survived much longer than American breast cancer patients, even those of Japanese ancestry.[3]

There are other cancer types with dismal survival rates. Lung cancer, for example, has a five-year survival rate of less than ten percent, meaning that fewer than one out of ten people are alive five years after their diagnosis. The Surgeon General's Report in 1979 reported that little significant progress in the diagnosis or treatment of lung cancer had been made in the previous fifteen years.[4] All that has changed since then is that the mortality rate of lung cancer in women surpassed that of breast cancer in 1987, clearly reflecting increased smoking rates among women.

Ovarian cancer has been correlated with the consumption of dairy products, particularly yogurt and cottage cheese. This was based on a study led by Daniel Cramer at Harvard University and published in *The Lancet* in 1989.[5] This and other studies show that dairy consumption increases the risk of lymphoma and leukemia as well.

If we could rule out two of the most preventable causes of cancers, smoking and high-fat diets, we would eliminate most of the cancers in this country and the West. The ones remaining, the relatively rare types of cancer, are the ones that are yielding to the new advances in cancer therapies. This is such an exciting thought that I wish had a magic wand and could just wave cigarettes and animal foods out of people's lives.

Given that this is impossible, there is an alternative that works: to make athletes out of all smokers and fat-eaters! Once a person starts an athletic training program and then starts competing in races, something that reinforces the training program, that person usually will not do those things that are counterproductive to winning.

This means that the person wins, the body wins, society wins, and nobody loses! There is no greater "high" than that of doing well in a race. And "well" doesn't necessarily mean placing first. For beginners, doing well means just finishing the race. For the more advanced, it means a PR (personal record), doing it faster than you've ever done it before. I've seen people jump up and down, scream, and generally just go crazy when they've set a new PR. It's that exciting for them.

There's also the joy of "first place," that excitement or pride that can last for years. Plus it's usually made more tangible by a neat trophy or plaque. Now this is not to say that success comes easy. There is discomfort, there's sometimes pain. There were times during the Ironman competitions that I felt extreme pain—pain so intense that I wondered why was putting myself through the agony.

But what I learned from earlier events was that all of a sudden the pain gets washed away with the euphoric joy of crossing that finish line. I never knew that it was anything but a feeling until I saw my first Ironman finish line photograph. I was astounded at the expression on my face. I had never seen a look so ecstatic. And it's been repeated with every finish line photo. There's just no substitute for the "high" this kind of success can give.

Scientists have postulated the feeling is caused by endorphins (chemicals the body makes that are similar to opiates) that make us feel good at times like that. Whether it's the endorphins or the purely intellectual joy of accomplishing a major goal is irrelevant. What is relevant is that psychologically there is a lot going on here, and it has to do with survival.

Why Some Make it and Some Don't

One of the great mysteries of cancer (and other diseases as well) is why some people survive when they are not expected to and some die who were expected to survive. Remember, in my case the doctors at first could not tell me whether I had three months, three years, or how long to live.

A theory promoted by the Simontons in their book *Getting Well Again* deals with this very subject.[6] It seems to boil down to whether or not the patient has the will to fight the disease. This will seems to be bolstered by visualization of the body's immune system actively engaging cancer cells in combat. As I was training over the hundreds of hours with my rhythmical paddling, pedaling, or plodding, I was probably in a state of self-hypnosis. I was giving myself suggestions about how I was getting stronger, healthier, and having my white blood cells kill cancer cells.

Visualization is a relatively passive process. You're supposed to sit or lie quietly and picture strong, powerful white blood cells searching and destroying confused, weak cancer cells. While working on it, I found myself gritting my teeth, trying to make the visualization more "real." I tried, through closed eyes, to "see" those white blood cells gobbling up vagrant cancer cells. All I really saw was a velvety purple with flashes here and there, as my squinting caused pressure on my optic nerve.

It was a different matter on the playing field, however. This was an active process. What an understatement to call doing an Ironman "active"! This was an entire day and part of a night spent swimming, biking, and running at race pace, feeling totally exhilarated, healthy, and in total control of my universe. These feelings for me are very real. No visualization is required. I'm on the move, attacking, in complete control of my life, and as far from passive as one can get.

As the feelings of fatigue start to creep up on me, I'm still battling on, except that now the "enemy" is real. My body is obeying all the commands to race for time in the senses of winning the race and winning in life. My body is functioning at its best while eating and drinking (that's part of the fun, too; I burn up around 10,000 calories doing an Ironman). I'm experiencing the full range of emotions, a microcosm of a lifetime, and gain a perspective of who I am and what I want out of life. That, I suppose, could be called "active visualization," since I feel my healthiest while competing.

Taking Control

All this has to be good for the immune system in the long run. In the short run, intense physical activity depresses the white blood cell count. For me, doing the Ironman was my way of taking control of my disease. Instead of doing nothing, or grasping at chemotherapy or radiation, I was being as active as I could possibly be. It's only a hypothesis at this point, but I feel that the feeling of loss of control when you are given the diagnosis of cancer is one of the deadliest aspects of this disease. And the only way I could counter that feeling and wrest control again was by setting my goal of doing an Ironman.

Over the years that I've been counseling cancer patients, I've observed that about twenty percent of people who are seriously ill would prefer to die if given the opportunity. About sixty percent of people are willing to live providing the doctor does the work and the treatment is not too uncomfortable. The final twenty percent say, "I'll do anything to get well. Just tell me what to do!"

This book and the program herein is written for people in that last category. It is also written for those who have not yet been diagnosed with a serious illness but, if they had been, would fall in that last category. People who follow this program will probably be successful in avoiding the two major preventable killers of Americans, heart disease and cancer. I hope you are in this group.

The discoveries I have made along this multi-year journey to the Ironman have been exciting and revolutionary. At first, the medical community was totally against the ideas that diet, exercise, and anything mental could possibly make a difference in the survival of a cancer patient. Little by little I was feeling my way. As I increased the exercise, I found my ability to take control was increasing. This also served as my psychological support. At the same time I started to see glimmerings in the press about the role of diet and exercise in the treatment of cancer patients.

About a year into this program, I got a letter from two Ohio State University researchers with a request to fill out a questionnaire about my exercise. They were onto the same thing I was. Another year went by and I got a phone call from a New York City (remember I'm in Hawaii) national running magazine reporter who'd heard about my unusual approach to dealing with cancer. That interview culminated in a very nice story on me which led to stories in *Newsday*, *USA Today*, *The Honolulu Star Bulletin*, *The Honolulu Advertiser*, and such international publications as the *New Zealand Herald*, Japan's *Asahi Shimbun*, Australia's running magazine *The Fun Runner*, and newspaper blurbs all over the U.S. and in Russia, Thailand, and Nepal. *Runner's World* magazine also presented me with their "Golden Shoe" award.

More recently, there have been even more positive results in the studies that have been carried out. Many different, recently published studies have suggested that regular exercise might reduce the risk of cancer. These studies show that non-active women had about twice the risk of breast cancer and almost three times the rate of cancer of the ovaries, uterus, cervix, and vagina.[7] Additionally, active women had about half the rate of lymphoma, leukemia, myeloma, Hodgkin's disease, and cancer of the thyroid. There were also much lower rates in the incidence of other, less frequent types of cancer.[8] While these studies are on the "before" side of the equation, it is clear to me that whatever prevents cancer logically will have a role in the control and spread of cancer once it's established in the body. Some oncologists believe that whatever initiates cancer also promotes cancer.

So, does my approach work? A study by C. Barber Mueller, M.D., showed that eighty-eight percent of the women who died following a diagnosis of cancer of the breast ultimately died of their breast cancer.[9] This was a study utilizing data collected for nineteen years by the Syracuse, N.Y. Upstate Medical Center Cancer Registry on 3,558 women. Since cancer cells can remain viable in vitro (in the laboratory) for up to fifty years, it's too soon to tell if my approach is working. Besides, an experiment of one is totally inadequate. What it can do, though, is point the way for others to try. We need more controlled studies to show that diet can make a difference in survival rates such as the studies that showed that women with breast cancer who changed to a low-fat diet have a longer disease-free interval.[10]

If you really want to live the "good" life, get "good food" and "good exercise," get yourself as fit as you can possibly be, or what I call "super-fit." Use the three-pronged approach of diet, exercise, and active visualization, and give it all you've got! It's a race worth winning!

Notes

Chapter One

1. U.S. Senate Select Committee on Nutrition and Human Needs. "Dietary Goals for the United States." (1987)
2. Wynder, E. "A Comparison of Survival Rates Between American and Japanese Patients with Breast Cancer," *Surg Gynecol Obstet* (1963) 117: 196
3. Wynder, E. The Dietary Environment and Cancer. *JAMA* (1977) 71:385-92
4. U.S. Dept. of Agriculture. "Nutritive value of foods." *HGB* (1981) 72

Chapter Three

1. Sabbagh, K. "The Psychopathology of Fringe Medicine", *The Skeptical Inquirer* (Winter 1985)
2. U.S. Dept. of Health, Education, and Welfare,` *Environmental Health Perspectives* (October 1979) 32
3. Willett, W. C, et al., "Dietary fat and fiber in relation to risk of breast cancer: An 8-year follow-up." *JAMA* (October 21 1992) 268 (15): 2037-44

Chapter Five

1. Burkitt, D., "Colon-rectal cancer: Fiber and other dietary factors." *Am J Clin Nutr* (1978) 31: 558-64
2. Horrobin, D. F., "The regulation of prostaglandin biosynthesis by manipulation of essential fatty acid metabolism." *Reviews in Pure and Applied Pharma-cological Sciences* (1983) 4: 339-83
3. Campbell, T. C., "A study on diet, nutrition, and disease in the People's Republic of China. Part 1." Division of Nutritional Sciences, Cornell University, Ithaca, NY, 1–8.
4. Harris, W. *The Scientific Basis of Vegetarianism.* Honolulu: Hawaii Health Pub-lishers (1995) 69-73
5. Heidrich, Ruth, Ph.D., *The Race for Life Cookbook.* Honolulu: Hawaii Health Pub-lishers (1994)

Chapter Six

1. Klatsky A. L., et al., "Coffee use prior to MI restudied: Heavier intake may increase the risk." *Am J Epid* (September 1990) 132: 479-88
2. Kiel, D. P., et al., "Caffeine and the Risk of Hip Fracture, the Framingham Study." *Am J Epid* (October 1990) 132:1675-85
3. Harvard University Study, quoted in *Longevity* Magazine (October 1989)
4. *Calcified Tissue International* (1992) 50:14-18
5. Marsh, A., "Cortical bone density of adult lacto-ovo vegetarian and omnivorous women." *J Am Diet Assn* (1980) 76:148-51
6. Nilsson, B. "Bone density in athletes." *Clin Orthop* (1971) 77: 170-82
7. Kanis, J. "Calcium supplementation of the diet-1: Not justified by present evidence." *Brit Med J* (1989) 298:137-149
8. Mazess, R. "Bone mineral content of North Alaskan Eskimos." *Amer J of Clin Nutr* (1974) 27: 916-925
9. Messina V. & Messina, M., *The Vegetarian Way: Total Health for You and Your Family.* New York: Crown (1996)
10. Rambeaut, P. "Skeletal changes during space flight." *The Lancet* (1985) ii: 1050-1052

Chapter Seven

1. McDougall, J. *McDougall's Medicine: A Challenging Second Opinion.* Piscataway, NJ: New Century Publishers (1985) 231-49
2. Kjeldsen-Dragh, J., et al., "Controlled trial of testing and one-year vegetarian diet in rheumatoid arthritis." *The Lancet* 338: (October 12, 1991) 899-902
3. Cooper, Kenneth, M.D., *Aerobics.* New York: Bantam Books (1968) 240-41

Chapter Eight

1. "Guidelines established for diet programs." *The Honolulu Advertiser* (February 10, 1999)

Chapter Nine

1. Francis, B. et al., "The Fitness Leader," *Human Kinetics*, Champaign IL (1989)

Chapter Eleven

1. "Effective Cycling." To find a location nearest you, contact the League of American Bicyclists, 1612 K Street NW, Suite 401, Washington DC 20006. Tel.: 202-822-1333, Fax: 202-822-1334. Website: www.bikeleague.org

Chapter Twelve

1. Cooper, *Aerobics.* op. cit.
2. Hill, D. W., et al, "Diurnal variations in responses to exercise of 'morning' types and 'evening' types." *Journal of Sports Med Phys Fitness* (September 1988) 28: 218-19
3. Beri, D. "Effect of dietary restrictions on disease activity in rheumatoid arthritis." *Ann Rheum Dis* (1988) 47:69-72

4. Inman, R. D., "Arthritis and Enteritis: An interface of protein manifestations." *Rheumatol* 14: 406-07, 198

5. Lane, N., "Long distance running, bone density, and osteoarthritis." *JAMA* (1986) 255: 1147-51

6. Aloia, J. "Prevention of involutional bone loss by exercise." *Ann Intern Med* (1978) 89: 356-58

7. Anderson, O., "Runner's World." (January 1998) 28

Chapter Fourteen

1. Winston, S., *Getting Organized*. New York: Warner Books (1980)

2. CareerTrack, "How to Organize Your Life & Get Rid of Clutter," 3085 Center Green Drive, Boulder CO 80301. Tel.: 1-800-334-6780

3. Rook, A., "An investigation into the longevity of Cambridge sportsmen." *Brit Med J* (1954) 8

4. Hoffman, J. *Hunza: Fifteen Secrets of the World's Healthiest and Oldest People*. Valley Center, CA: Professional Press Publishing Co., (1979)

Chapter Fifteen

1. Hirayama, T. "Epidemiology of prostate cancer with special reference to the role of the diet." *JNCI Monogr* (1979) 53:149-55

2. Lee, J., "Natural Progesterone: The Multiple Roles of a Remarkable Hormone." *BLL Publishing* (1995)

3. Ibid., 3

4. Chang, K. J., et al., "Influences of percutaneous administration of estradiol and progesterone on human breast epithelial cell cycle in vivo." *Fertility and Sterility* (1995) 63: 785-91

5. Henig, R. *How A Woman Ages*. New York: Ballantine Books (1985)

6. Whitten, P. *The Complete Book of Swimming*. New York: Random House (1994)

Chapter Sixteen

1. Mares-Perlman, J. A. "Contribution of Epidemiology to Understanding Relations of Diet to Age-related Cataract." *Am J of Clin Nutr* (October 1997) 66: 739-40

2. Mayne, S., "Beta-carotene, Carotenoids, and Disease Prevention in Humans." *FASEBJ* (May 10 1996): 690-701

Chapter Seventeen

1. Holtzmuller, K. Personal communication. (July 1990)

Chapter Twenty

1. Carroll, K. "Experimental Evidence of Dietary Factors and Hormone Depen-dent Cancer." *Cancer Research* (1975) 35: 3374

2. Lowenthals, A.B., et al., "Diet and Cancer," *Cancer* (April 1977) 39 (4 Suppl): 1809-14

3. Wynder, E., "A Comparison of Survival Rates Between American and Japa-nese Patients with Breast Cancer." *Surg Gynecol Obstet* 117 (1963):196

4. Surgeon General's Report, "Clinical Implications of Surgeon General's Report on Smoking and Health." *J Nat Med Assoc* (July 1979) 71: 713-15

5. Cramer, D., et al., "Galactose Consumption and Metabolism in Relation to the Risk of Ovarian Cancer." *The Lancet* (July 8 1989) 66-71

6. Simonton, O. C. et al., *Getting Well Again.* New York: J. P. Tarcher, Inc. (1978)

7. Frisch, R., "Lower prevalence of breast cancer and cancers of the reproduc-tive system among former college athletes compared to non-athletes." *Br J Cancer* (1985) 52: 885-91

8. Kohl, H. "Physical activity and cancer: An epidemiological perspective." *Sports Medicine* (1988) 6: 222-37

9. Mueller, C. B. et al., "Breast cancer in 3558 women: Age as a significant determinant in the rate of dying and causes of death." *Surgery* (February 1978) 123, 83:2.

10. Holm, L. E., et al., "Treatment Failure and Dietary Habits in Women With Breast Cancer." J National Cancer Institute (January 6 1993) 85:1

Resources

Books

Bailey, Covert. *Fit Or Fat*. Boston: Houghton Mifflin (1978)

Barnard, Neal, M.D.. *Foods That Fight Pain: Revolutionary New Strategies for Maximum Pain Relief*. New York: Avon (1999)

———. *Food for Life: How the New Four Food Groups Can Save Your Life*. New York: Crown Publishing Group (1994)

———. *The Power of Your Plate: Eating Well for Better Health—20 Experts Tell You How!* Summertown, TN: Book Publishing Company (1996)

Borysewicz, Edward. *Bicycle Road Racing*. Brattleboro, VT: Velo-News Corp (1985)

Cooper, Kenneth, M.D. *Aerobics*. New York: Bantam Books (1968)

Harris, W., M.D. *The Scientific Basis of Vegetarianism*. Honolulu: Hawaii HealthPublishers (1995)

Henig, Robin. *How A Woman Ages*. New York: Ballantine Books (1985)

Keon, Joseph, Ph.D. *The Truth About Breast Cancer: A 7 Step Prevention Plan*. Mill Valley, CA: Parissound Publishing (1999)

Klaper, Michael, M.D. *Vegan Nutrition: Pure and Simple*. Umatilla, FL: Gentle World (1997)

Kradjian, Robert M., M.D. *Save Yourself from Breast Cancer*. New York: Berkley Publishing (1994)

Lee, John, M.D. *Natural Progesterone: The Natural Way to Alleviate Symptoms of Menopause, PMS, and Other Hormone Related Problems*. Sebastopol, CA: BLL Publishing (1994)

McDougall, John, M.D. *The McDougall Program: Twelve Days to Dynamic Health*. New York: Plume (1991)

———. *McDougall's Medicine: A Challenging Second Opinion*. Clinton, NJ: New Win Publishing (1986)

———. *The McDougall Program for Maximum Weight Loss*. New York: Dutton (1994)

McDougall, John, M.D and Mary McDougall. *The McDougall Program for Women: What Every Woman Needs to Be Healthy for Life*. New York: Dutton (1999)

——. *The McDougall Plan:* Clinton, NJ: New Win Publishing (1985)

——. *The McDougall Program for a Healthy Heart: A Life-Saving Approach to Pre-venting and Treating Heart Disease.* New York: Plume (1998)

——. *The New McDougall Cookbook.* New York: Plume (1997)

McDougall, Mary. *The McDougall Health-Supporting Cookbook, Vols 1 & 2* Clinton, NJ: New Win Publishing (1985, 1986)

The McDougall Newsletter, P.O. Box 14039, Santa Rosa, CA 95402.

Morra, Marion, and Eve Potts. *Choices: Realistic Alternatives in Cancer Treatment.* New York: Avon (1994)

Notelovitz, Morris, M.D, and Marsha Ware. *Stand Tall!: Every Woman's Guide to Preventing and Treating Osteoporosis.* Gainesville, FL: Triad Publishing (1998)

Ornish, Dean, M.D. *Dr. Dean Ornish's Program for Reversing Heart Disease.* New York: Random House (1995)

——. *Eat More, Weigh Less: Dr. Dean Ornish's Life Choice Program for Losing Weight Safely.* San Francisco: Harper San Francisco (1997)

Ostrander, Sheila, and Lynn Schroeder. *Superlearning.* New York: Dell Publishing (1979)

Prins Jan, Ph.D. *The Illustrated Swimmer.* Honolulu, HI: He'e (1982)

Robbins, John. *Diet For A New America: How Your Food Choices Affect Your Health, Happiness, and the Future of Life on Earth.* Tiburon, CA: H. J. Kramer (1998)

——. *May All Be Fed: A Diet for A New World.* New York: Avon (1993)

——. *Reclaiming Our Health: Exploding the Medical Myth and Embracing the Sources of True Healing.* Tiburon, CA: H. J. Kramer (1998)

Scott, Dave. *David Scott's Triathlon Training.* New York: Simon & Schuster (1986)

Siegel, Bernie, M.D. *Love, Medicine & Miracles: Lessons Learned about Self-Healing from a Surgeon's Experience with Exceptional Patients.* New York: Harper & Row (1986)

Simonton, O. Carl, M.D, and Stephanie Matthews-Simonton. *Getting Well Again.* New York: Tarcher (1978)

Organizations and Periodicals

American Cancer Society Reach to Recovery Program, 777 Third Ave., New York, NY 10017

American Vegan Society, P.O. Box H. Malaga, NJ 08328

Bicycling Magazine, Box 7308, Red Oak, IA 51591

EarthSave International, 444 NE Ravenna Blvd, Suite 205, Seattle, WA 98105. Tel.: 206-524-9903. Web site: www.earthsave.org

Effective Cycling, League of American Bicyclists, 1612 K St., Suite 401, Wash-ington DC 20006. Tel.: 202-822-1333. Web site: www.bikeleague.org

Ruth Heidrich's Web site: www.ironlady.com

Institute of Nutrition Education and Research, 1601 N. Sepulveda Blvd., Suite 342, Manhattan Beach, CA 90266. Tel.: 310-374-3733. Web site: www.vegsource. com/ klaper/institute.htm

International Vegetarian Union, P.O. Box 9710, Washington, DC 20016. Tel.: 202-362-VEGY, Box 3. Web site: www.ivu.org

McDougall Wellness Center, P.O. Box 14039, Santa Rosa, CA 95402. Tel.: 800-570-1654. Web site: www.drmcdougall.com

North American Vegetarian Society, P.O. Box 72 Dolgeville, NY 13329. Tel.: 518-568-7970. Email: navs@telenet.org; Web site: www.navs_online.org

A Race for Life Video and *A Race for Life Cookbook*, 1415 Victoria St. #1106, Hono-lulu, HI 96822

Road Runner's Club of America, RRCA National Office, 1150 South Washington Street, Suite 250, Alexandria, VA 22314-4493. Tel.: 703-836-0558. Web site: www.rrca.org

Runner's World Magazine, P.O. Box 7307, Red Oak, IA 51591-0307. Tel.: 800-666-2828. Web site: www.runnersworld.com

Running Network, 7840 N. Lincoln Ave. Suite 208, Skokie, IL 60077. Tel.:847-675-0200. Web site: www.runningnetwork.com

Satya: A Magazine of Vegetarianism, Environmentalism, and Animal Advocacy, P.O. Box 138, New York, NY 10012. Tel.: 212-674-0952. Web site: www.stealth- technolo-gies.com/satya

Swim Magazine, 228 Nevada St., El Segundo, CA 90245

Vegan Outreach, 211 Indian Drive, Pittsburgh, PA 15238. Tel.: 412-968-0268. Web site: www.veganoutreach.org

Vegetarian Resource Group, P.O. Box 1463, Baltimore, MD 21203. Tel.: 410-366-8343. Web site: www.vrg.org

Vegetarian Times, 4 High Ridge Park, Stamford, CT 06908. Tel.: 203-322-2900. Web site: www.vegetariantimes.com

Vegsource: The On-Line Resource for Vegetarianism: www.vegsource.org

VivaVegie Society, P.O. Box 294, Prince Street Station, New York, NY 10012. Tel.: 212-591-2914. Web site: www.vivavegie.org

Voice for a Viable Future, 11288 Ventura Blvd., #202A, Studio City, CA 91604. Tel.: 818-509-1255. Web site: www.madcowboy.com

Seven-Day Meal Plan

MONDAY
Breakfast: Oatmeal with Apple Juice* Orange Sections
Lunch: Pho (Vietnamese Soup)*
Dinner: Rice Ramen Curry*

TUESDAY
Breakfast: Buckwheat Cereal with Cranberry Juice
Lunch: Vegetarian Sandwich*
Dinner: Spaghetti Marinara with Tossed Green Salad

WEDNESDAY
Breakfast: Wheat Berries with Mango Juice*
Lunch: Texas Fries, Apple and Pear Slices*
Dinner: Pizza*

THURSDAY
Breakfast: Grape Nuts with Apple Juice
Lunch: Fruit Sandwich*
Dinner: Baked Squash with Brown Rice and Broccoli

FRIDAY
Breakfast: Shredded Wheat with Guava Juice
Lunch: Split Pea Soup*
Dinner: Lentil Loaf with Corn on the Cob*

SATURDAY

Breakfast: Pancakes with Applesauce*
Lunch: Baked Potato with Salsa
Dinner: Wild Rice with Beets and Brussel Sprouts

SUNDAY

Breakfast: Waffles with Strawberries*
Lunch: Stuffed Pita Bread Sandwich
Dinner: Eggplant Szechwan with Brown Rice*

* see recipes

Recipes

Two-Minute Oatmeal

 1/2 c. old-fashioned rolled oats
 1 banana
 1 tsp. Blackstrap molasses
 Water to cover

Pour oatmeal into cereal bowl and add water. Microwave for two minutes or eat as is. Add sliced banana, molasses, or any combination of fruit.

Pho (Vietnamese Soup)

 1 cup cooked brown rice
 1 sm. pkg. Nori (seaweed)
 1/2 bunch chopped parsley
 1 T. miso
 1–2 c. water (to top off bowl)
 1/2 tsp. hot chili sauce (to taste)
 1/2 bunch beet greens, cabbage, or other greens

Add all ingredients to large soup bowl and microwave for four minutes. Stir thoroughly.

Rice Ramen Curry

 1 pot cooked brown rice
 1 c. Chinese parsley, chopped
 1 pkg. low-fat ramen noodles
 1 T. curry powder
 1/2 c. raisins

Cook brown rice. While rice is cooking, break up the ramen noodles while still in package with the heel of the hand until there are no large chunks. Open package, remove spice package, and mix crushed noodles with the cooked brown rice. (The heat of the rice "cooks" the noodles.) Add the spice packet, curry powder, parsley, and raisins. Ready to serve hot or cold.

Vegetarian Sandwich

> Assorted sliced veggies, e.g., Romaine, kale, tomato, cucumber, sprouts, etc.
> 2 slices whole grain bread or pita

Arrange sliced veggies between slices of bread or in pita pocket. Add condiments if desired.

Wheat Berries

Cook wheat berries until soft, or the night before pour wheat berries into a thermos of boiling water and cover overnight. Add fruit and serve. This technique works with all types of whole grains.

Texas Fries

> 2-3 potatoes, any type

Cut into lengthwise quarters and microwave approximately seven to ten minutes, depending on size. They taste great just plain, but you can sprinkle vinegar, garlic powder, paprika, or other herbs on them.

Pizza

> Pita bread
> 1 T. oregano
> 1 can tomato sauce or 1/2 c. salsa
> 1 T. basil
> Veggies, e.g., bell pepper slices, mushrooms, chopped onions, sprouts, etc.

Spread veggies on split pita bread. Bake or microwave until bubbly. If a "cheese" topping is desired, sprinkle nutritional yeast on top.

Fruit Sandwich

> Assorted fruits
> Pita or other whole grain bread

Arrange slices of fruit in pita pockets or on bread slices.

Split Pea Soup

> 2 c. split peas
> 1 onion, chopped
> 2 qt. water
> pinch cayenne
> 4 ribs diced celery
> 1 bay leaf
> 2 carrots, diced
> 1/2 tsp. thyme

Combine all ingredients in a large pot, bring to boil and simmer one hour, or four hours in a slow cooker.

Lentil Loaf

2 c. cooked lentils
1 can tomato sauce
1 chopped onion
1 c. rolled oats, uncooked
Herbs: garlic, parsley, basil, oregano, fennel, etc

Preheat oven to 350 degrees F. Combine all ingredients, mixing well. Put into eight by four by two inch loaf pan. Bake forty-five minutes.

Pancakes or Waffles

2 c. whole wheat flour
1 T. blackstrap molasses
1 c. rolled oats
1 T. baking powder
3 c. water
1 T. each vanilla and cinnamon

Combine ingredients in a medium bowl, taking care not to over-mix. Preheat griddle on medium high for about five minutes or until a drop of water dances on the griddle, or about ten minutes on the waffle iron. Spray surface with non-stick cooking spray. Ladle batter onto griddle or iron. Turn pancakes when bubbles appear and give them another minute or so. Waffles are ready when the steam stops rising from the iron, about a minute and a half. Do not open the waffle iron too soon or the waffle will separate. Use desired fruit topping such as strawberries, preserves, or applesauce.

Eggplant Szechwan

2-3 eggplants
2 T. low-sodium soy sauce
1 green onion, sliced
1 T. cornstarch
1 tsp. chili sauce, or to taste
2 c. water
1 T. ginger, minced and preferably fresh

Slice eggplant. Put in a large, round casserole dish. Add cornstarch to water, mixing well. Add with remaining ingredients to eggplant and bake. If in microwave, about five to six minutes, or in conventional oven, about twenty-five minutes at 350 degrees F.

Appendix One

Interpretation of Labratory Tests

The following information is provided as a quick reference so you can look up the results of your lab tests. Since there are variations between laboratories, this information is not guaranteed to be accurate. Use this as a rough guide to learn more about lab tests and what information they provide about your body. The bracketed figures are ideal rates. Measurement abbreviations are as follows: mg (milligrams), dl (deciliter or a tenth of a liter), μl (microliter or one millionth of a liter), meq (milli equivalents or a thousand parts), mcg (micrograms or one millionth of a gram), ng (nanograms or one billionth of a gram), μmol (micromoles or one millionth of the molecular weight).

CHOL (100–160 mg/dl): stands for blood cholesterol. This is probably the most important of all the blood tests. If you are average (220 mg/dl) then you have an average risk for heart attack (better than 50 percent), breast cancer (1 in 9 for women), colon cancer (1 in 20), and gallbladder disease (1 in 5). Cholesterol is found only in animal products, and conversely all animal products contain cholesterol. Our own bodies make all the cholesterol we need. When we eat additional cholesterol in the form of animal products, it is readily absorbed. The problem develops because our livers can only break down a limited amount of this substance per day. The excess accumulates in body tissues like arteries, skin, organs, and body fat. Your blood level reflects the level of cholesterol in your body. The ideal level is 160 mg/dl or less. Replacing animal foods with starches, vegetables, and fruits will cause the cholesterol to fall 30-100 mg/dl in most people in fewer than 21 days. Maintenance of this diet will result in continued improvement.

Excreted cholesterol enters the gallbladder, thereby contributing to gallstones (90 percent are made of cholesterol). Cholesterol in the colon is believed to be involved in colon cancer. Eating vegetable oils will cause more cholesterol to be excreted with a rise in a person's risk of gallbladder disease and colon cancer. A change to a no-cholesterol diet is the most effective and safest way to lower your cholesterol. All plant foods contain no cholesterol. Coconuts and chocolate contain enough saturated fat to raise cholesterol levels in the blood.

HDL *(Male 26–66 mg/dl; Female 30–75 mg/dl):* stands for High Density Lipoprotein, a fraction of the total cholesterol with some predictive value for risk of heart disease. HDL is an end product of cholesterol metabolism and represents the cholesterol that is leaving the tissues on the way to being excreted by the liver. If your level is low and you're consuming the typical American diet, you should consider this an indication that it's time to start a low/no cholesterol diet. People on low cholesterol diets have low HDL because of the low total cholesterol.

GLUCOSE (65–120 mg/dl): the sugar in your blood. When you haven't eaten for a while, the level is normally between 65 and 120 mg/dl. When the body loses control of sugar levels, the condition is called diabetes (levels over 120 mg/dl). Most diabetes (95 percent) is the so-called adult-onset Type II, and is caused by a high fat, low-fiber diet. Correction of the diet will solve this problem for most people. Exercise and weight loss also help. Type I, childhood-onset diabetes, is a different condition that results from destruction of portions of the pancreas that produce insulin. While diet will not cure this type, a proper diet will certainly help. Hypoglycemia is a condition of low blood sugar (below 50 mg/dl). Another test (the five-hour glucose tolerance test) is used to make this diagnosis. The cause and correction are diet.

BUN *(6–25 mg/dl):* stands for Blood Urea Nitrogen, the breakdown products of protein. BUN is made in the liver and excreted by the kidneys. Low protein diets lower BUN. Kidney disease can cause the BUN to rise and make people feel ill.

CREA *(0.7–1.4 mg/dl):* stands for creatinine, a breakdown product from muscle, excreted by the kidneys. Elevation usually means kidney disease.

URIC ACID *(2.2–7.7 mg/dl):* a breakdown product of purines which are found in high protein foods such as meat, seafood, chicken, cheese, and beans. Large amounts of uric acid can lead to gout (arthritis) and kidney stones.

TRIG *(50–275 mg/dl):* stands for triglycerides, blood fats. If your blood were to stand in a test tube overnight, a layer of fat would rise to the top. High levels are associated with heart attacks, diabetes, and poor circulation which result in chest pain, leg pain, and fatigue. Triglycerides are elevated by consuming alcoholic beverages, simple sugars, and fats. Even fruit and fruit juice can elevate the levels in sensitive people. Exercise, high fiber foods, and weight loss will lower triglycerides to healthy levels. Note that sometimes during a period of weight loss, triglycerides may temporarily rise due to the movement of fat from the fat tissues to the blood. You should try to keep your levels below 200 mg/dl.

BILI *(1.1–1.7 mg/dl):* a breakdown product of red blood cells. It is elevated when there is a large breakdown of blood cells, and when the liver is diseased and unable to adequately excrete it. Many people have a slight elevation (up to 3 mg/dl) that may occur as a result of overnight fasting. The best indication of normal is that all the other liver tests are normal.

SGOT *(7–50 μl),* **SGPT** *(7–50 μl),* **LDH** *(90–225 μl):* abbreviations for liver enzymes that are released when the liver is injured. Gallbladder disease, excess alcohol consumption, and viruses causing hepatitis are the most common causes of elevation.

ALK PHOS *(30–115 μl):* stands for alkaline phosphatase, an enzyme from either the bones or the liver. It can be elevated in bone or gallbladder disease.

INORG P *(2.0–4.7 mg/dl):* stands for inorganic phosphorus. Levels increase with amount of phosphorus in your diet.

CALCIUM *(8.8–10.8 mg/dl):* a mineral with many functions in the body. Blood levels must be kept at minimum critical levels. Therefore, calcium levels are almost always normal. Abnormal values usually reflect laboratory error or a decrease in the albumin protein in the blood, due to liver or kidney disease. The level of calcium in your blood does not reflect the amount of calcium in your diet or in your bones.

NA *(135–145 meq/l):* stands for sodium, a mineral found in large quantities in the body. The level does not reflect your dietary intake of salt. Sometimes the level is low when people are taking diuretics, or medications to lower blood pressure.

K *(3.5–5.5 meq/l):* stands for potassium, a mineral also found in large amounts in the body. Levels do not reflect dietary intake unless you have serious kidney disease. Sometimes the level is low when people are on diuretics. This mineral must be kept in the normal range or death can result.

CL *(96–110 meq/l)* and **CO^2** *(25–32 meq/l):* stands for chlorine and carbon dioxide, usually at normal levels in the blood unless people are on medications.

TOT PRO *(6.2–8.3 g/dl):* stands for total protein which represents the protein floating in the blood. These proteins are made primarily by the liver and the immune system. They may be elevated in certain infections and disease of the bone marrow.

ALBUMIN *(3.6–5.2 g/dl):* a protein made in the liver, down in serious liver and kidney disease.

GLOBULIN *(2.5 g/dl):* the protein made by the immune system for defense.

A/G *(1.1-2.2): stands for the ratio of albumin to globulin.*

HEMOGLOBIN *(Male 14–18 g/dl; Female 12–16 g/dl):* the oxygen-carrying, red-pigmented, iron-containing substance in the blood. The level reflects the amount of red blood cells in the body, and a low level can mean anemia. Twenty percent of women in this country have iron deficiency anemia. Dairy products contribute to this problem in several ways. Cow's milk is deficient in iron, and the calcium and phosphorus in cow's milk complexes iron from other sources to prevent absorption. The fats in dairy products and other foods cause higher levels of estrogen in a woman's body with resulting heavier menstrual periods with more blood loss each month. Anyone with anemia should be checked for blood loss in their stools at the minimum.

HCT *(40–55 percent, slightly lower in women):* Hematocrit shows the percentage of blood cells (mostly red blood cells) comprising the total blood volume. Used as a test for anemia and dehydration, and to follow the course of therapy for anemia.

TIBC *(200–400 mcg/100 ml):* stands for Total Iron-binding Capacity and is usually increased only with an iron-deficiency anemia, a type of anemia usually associated with blood loss.

SERUM FERRITIN *(30 ng/100 ml and up):* a measure of the iron stores in the body. Decreased ferritin is found with iron deficiency but not with an anemia of infection. Increased ferritin is found with excessive iron intake.

Homosysteine *(5–15 μmol/l),* an amino acid associated with vascular disease. [Please note different notation for "umol"]

Glossary

Aerobic Integrity: A level of oxygen-burning exercise at which the body can maintain a sustained output for an extended period of time without going into oxygen debt.

Amnesia: Lack or loss of memory. **Anterograde a.,** loss of memory for events which occurred after the onset of the disease. **Retrograde a.,** loss of memory for events which occurred before the onset of the disease.

Anaerobic: An inability to maintain an oxygen level in the body to support continued exercise. Leads to oxygen debt.

Anemia: Deficient quantity or quality of the blood. Usually marked by paleness and fatigue.

Areola: The pigmented area surrounding the nipple.

Biathlon: Any two-sport race, for example, a swim–run, or a bike–run.

Biceps: The large flexor muscle of the front of the upper arm.

Biopsy: Examination of tissue removed from a living subject.

Carbohydrates: Starchy and sugary foods; compounds made up of carbon in groups of six atoms, and hydrogen and oxygen in proportions to form water. Have four calories/g.

Chemotherapy: Treatment by powerful chemical compounds which have a toxic effect on specific cells or micro-organisms. Cancer cells, which are frequently weak and disorganized, are usually more vulnerable to the effects of this treatment.

Cholesterol: A waxy substance produced in the liver of all animals. Makes up the structural integrity of all animal cells.

Endorphins: Chemicals produced by the body which create pleasant feelings. Contributes to the so-called "runner's high."

Epidemiology: The branch of science that deals with the occurrence, distribution, and types of diseases; population studies.

Fascia: the band or sheet of connective tissue covering the muscles.

Fat: The oily substance that covers the connective tissues of animals; an organic salt consisting of the glycerol radical, C_3H_5, combined with a fatty acid. Has more than twice the number of calories of carbohydrate and protein, nine calories/g.

Hydrostatic body fat test: A method of estimating percent of body fat by immersion in water.

Infiltrating ductal carcinoma: Moderately metastasizing, invasive breast cancer accounting for about sixty-five percent of all breast cancers. May spread to liver, lungs, bones, and brain. Usually cannot be eradicated by local treatment of breast and lymph nodes. Usually has spread to bloodstream by the time clinical symptoms are evident.

Lacto-ovo-vegetarian: A person who avoids all animal products except dairy products and eggs. This diet will still be high in animal fat and cholesterol. Milk has been referred to as "liquid meat."

LASIK (Laser-assisted in situ keratomileusis) which corrects vision by changing the shape of the cornea. A hinged flap is cut on the surface of the cornea and a laser reshapes the underlying corneal tissue, which corrects vision by changing the shape of the cornea.

Liposuction: A surgical procedure whereby fat is sucked out of the body in very specific areas.

Marathon: A footrace of 26.2 miles. Originated in Greece in 490 B.C. When the Athenians defeated the Persians, a messenger, Phidipides, was sent to bear the news of the victory to Athens. The name is derived from his run starting at the battle-site of Marathon. Now, most cities and countries of the world conduct these races annually.

Mastectomy: The surgical amputation of the breast; **modified radical m.** removal of breast plus skin, nipple, subcutaneous fat, fascia, and axillary (armpit) nodes; **simple m.** removal of breast tissue only, leaving skin and nipple; **radical m.** removal of breast, skin, nipple, fascia, subcutaneous fat, axillary nodes, and the pectoral (chest) muscles; **lumpectomy:** removal of the tumor and a margin of healthy tissue surrounding tumor.

Metastasis: Spread of disease from one organ to another. Cancerous cells break off from the primary tumor and invade the bloodstream or lymphatics. Once there, these cells travel to other parts of the body, such as the lungs, liver, bones, and brain, setting up new cancerous tumor colonies.

Oncology, -ist: The study of tumors and cancers and the person who studies them.

Osteoporosis: The thinning or abnormal porpusness of the bones, the cause of which is still debated. Most recent studies show that the best treatment, as well as prevention, is exercise and a low protein diet.

Protein: Combinations of amino acids and their derivatives found in animal and vegetable tissues. Has four calories/g.

Reconstructive breast surgery: The insertion of an implant under the skin to restore the normal body contours when lost due to an amputated breast. Nipples and areolae may also be reconstructed by using various body parts such as earlobes, skin from the upper inner thigh, etc.

Subcutaneous: Under the skin. May refer to implant placement when used in reconstructive breast surgery as opposed to sub-muscular, under the chest muscle.

Triathlon: Any three-sport race; conventionally, a swim, bike, run.

Ultramarathon: Any footrace longer than a marathon (26.2 miles).

Vegan: A vegetarian diet that is devoid of all animal products, including dairy products and eggs. Biochemically, there is very little difference in the composition of meat, dairy products, and eggs. All animal products are high in fat, high in cholesterol, and low in fiber and iron.